CAMOUFLAGING CORONA

SAJIKUMAR

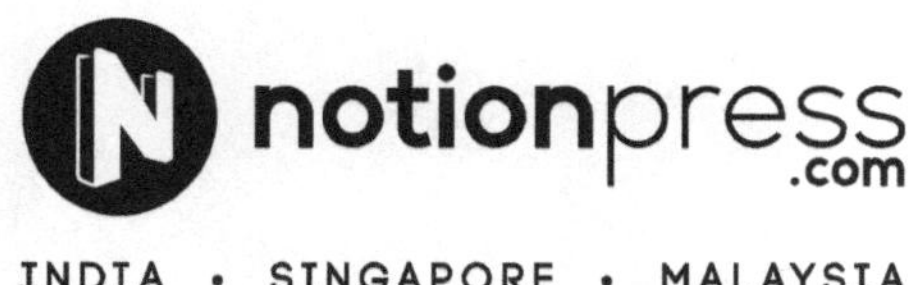

INDIA • SINGAPORE • MALAYSIA

ISBN 979-8-89277-921-0

Contents

Preface

One of the famous British scientists commented at the time of Covid-19 that in case we put the complete coronavirus in a Coca-Cola bottle, it cannot be filled. Just imagine this; he has not mentioned the quantity required to infect a single person but the 13-crore people who got infected and were affected by Covid-19. Just imagine such a small quantity of viruses threatening us.

But more than the virus, the name of the virus created much damage to humanity. Death from disease is unnatural, and if we could accept this as a fact, we could have minimised the damage.

If we believe that viruses create damage, then we should know more about the virus and their presence in our body, whether they are helping, troubling, or balancing the system.

The scientists believed that science had grown up to new heights, but I believe there is less study on microorganisms and scientists should learn more about microorganisms. Instead of finding out better or correct, they focus on proving themselves or see where there is more commercial benefit. They are not concerned about the rest. They are taking advantage of a layman's knowledge. In recent years, science has identified various viruses and studied them. The world of viruses is small compared to any other microorganisms. But their number is very huge. So, viruses can not only benefit us but can also damage us. When a virus is threatened in its environment, it reacts positively or adversely, and that causes trouble for us.

Science says that microbes are necessary, and they are everywhere; those fungi, viruses, and bacteria are giving us life. If microbes are everywhere, we can't stop them from entering our noses or any part of our body. So, I must say scientists were fooling us by giving us much advice, but we have no courage to say it loudly. And unfortunately, the same system has asked us to wear a mask to protect against the tiny viruses, and we are obliged even when science says that these microbes are living everywhere.

According to certain scientists, the human body carries 370 billion viruses, and it only carries 37 billion bacteria. Still, no one can find out the exact number of microbes and their varieties. Yet, they are good at concluding everything by assuming.

Viruses are no danger like we think; if so, they could damage the entire living system, instead, they help in many ways to continue life. Science is aware of that, as every kind of change that has happened in the human body is a contribution of viruses. Viruses are instrumental in forming our placenta, females to conceiving, creating sexual interest, delivering babies, wound healing, and many other things. Viruses are working, they are living, and they have a helpful hand in human systems, and that is a fact.

Human interference like migration and other things has created an aggressive change in the viruses. In the process, certain kinds of viruses have become very dangerous because we started to use uncontrolled antibiotics for animal growth. Otherwise, viruses were unharming living within their ecosystem.

Viruses have always helped us, and we humans are the culprits. The human body has 10% of the virus genes, showing they are primitive, like our first parents-our ancestors and we humans, in turn, always wanted to wash out the bitter truth.

Through evolution, we have changed through many lives, so when we wish to read about our ancestors, it is better to read about chimpanzees; our history must be the same. Interestingly, almost every primitive human, including chimpanzees, are carrying the same virus gene.

If we were to calculate the total number of virus genes in our body, the number of virus genes in our body would be very high, and we are like one of their homes. So, they can enter our bodies very easily because it belongs to them too. Thus, next time when we proudly say 'I,' we should realise there is nothing called 'me' or 'I' in us.

Outside of the human body, in all kinds of life—all trees, plants, animals—all kinds of life—there are bacteria and viruses; they work everywhere for themselves and us, so we can live our lives.

In that case, we can say they are the masters and not we humans. Because of them, we are living, mating, having children, breathing, eating, and thinking, all of these things are not possible when viruses do not exist.

Imagine when COVID-19 was declared by the WHO. They forced us to use sanitiser, wash our hands, and wear masks, but I am surprised why such a big organisation sees only human interest.

In that case, just imagine: if viruses are everywhere in the world and viruses are the only thing giving life, and viruses are only supporting the living system, then how can we prevent viruses?

Knowing this fact, the authorities forcefully administered vaccination. Science could have given a better explanation to people about microbes, and we could have dealt with the pandemic in a better way.

Chapter 1

A Branded Viral Disease Called Covid-19

If the viral disease that appeared in 1976 was named Ebola to signify the name of an African river where it originated, Covid-19 should have been named Wuhan.

U.S. FDA approved a vaccine for Ebola in 2019, the year the COVID-19 pandemic emerged. Ebola ended in 2020 giving a gentle space for Covid-19, which was named brilliantly with a number to recall the year it started, to leave a mark on humankind.

From the beginning of the Covid-19 pandemic, there were many things suspicious. Soon, the scenario started unveiling a near-true picture. For any product, naming is very important, and like any major disease, this was given a good brand name too. The architect of the pandemic plot was aware, none would question their plot, and they can promote it under a serious name. Thus, a crime against humanity remained unquestioned.

It is unheard of and absurd to imagine. It may even be construed as an overzealous attack on health organisations and the medical world. But it is true with the name of Covid-19; whoever named it did it brilliantly. The naming was done creatively making it universally pronounceable and uniformly articulate.

It is after all a flu but was named differently to build it as a brand. None would dare ask doctors, medical scientists, and virologists about the logic, and none could refuse to accept what would be offered as a justification. It was unusual to see a disease named after the common English word- virus. A perfectly recallable and catchy name that would make its marketing easier. The creator of the disease visualised their big empire developing over a period.

None of the scientists wanted to call the disease flu. The virus is not new to the human body, but China reported it for the first time under much suspense and fear, and the world saw it as deadly and fearful. By the time the world considered COVID-19 deadly, China had convinced the world of Covid's danger and could control it back home. However, the world was made to believe in impending fears.

Yet, when the World Health Organisation (WHO) came out with its interpretation, the United States expressed displeasure over WHO's soft corner with China.

The disease was baptised as Covid-19 – a short form of coronavirus Disease with the year of its emergence, which is 2019.

However, the naming was a deviation from the history of human diseases. Most diseases were named in European classical languages, except Ebola, which was named after an African river from where it emerged. Going by the nomenclature of Ebola, Covid-19 should have been named Wuhan-19.

The name flu, derived from the word influenza, has now become generic. A deviated name meant a new space, for which phobia could be created by terming it novel. A new virus and a new and impactful propaganda. The brand can thus imprint fear and affect people's psyches.

Thus, a brand called COVID-19 was created that appeared on every page of newspapers and occupied billions of bytes of online media, in turn threatening mankind.

Rich countries and medical Czars fuelled their ambition to make a business from this brand and rule the world of infected people. They spent trillions, initially to own patents and intellectual property rights for vaccine development. In all this, looking at the probable beneficiaries of the brand, let the world never forget China.

The human world pays heavily to the multiple beneficiaries of a single global brand. Many of the celebrated global organisations, which provide first-line disaster response service, as aides to the state authorities around the world, did not comment on the spread of the disease. Though the philanthropic organisations might have done their work, many a time, they too were not free from suspicion.

After India kept silent on China's offer of aid, the Red Cross Society of China sent oxygen concentrators, ventilators, and cash of $1 million to the Indian Red Cross Society through the International Federation of Red Cross and Red Crescent Societies. Aids came from around the world without India asking for any aid, as a gesture of gratitude. The world is aware that India is a big market for every trade.

Chapter 2

Inside the Blanket of Infection

Who expected a pandemic? Who envisaged the way things turned out and how the world was swept by an unprecedented deadly disease? While the pandemic has left trailing destruction, the full extent of it cannot be calculated or estimated through human lives lost and economic downfall. The pandemic was just the tip of the iceberg, and what we all have to come to terms with now is the massive chunk that remains underwater, unseen and unestimated.

The aftermath of every world event is not just the economic turmoil, but the mental deluge that survives in each mind like a ticking time bomb.

With Covid-19, financial losses, loss of jobs, loss of dear ones, vulnerability to experimental medication, and all its aftereffects are compounded and etched deep in people's minds. Race, ethnicity, location, culture, age, status, or religion, every human has lasting impressions of the pandemic.

Around early 2020, the pandemic news was faintly heard in international news. It all started surfacing prominently in Indian news channels only in early March 2020. A rare kind of viral infection has been found amongst the people in China's Wuhan wet market. The news was on the corners and inside pages of broadsheets and had to still hit the front page. Indian media did not pay much heed in the early days, as China claimed the scope and extent of the virus, and WHO vouched for the same. The media perhaps did not estimate the intensity of the marketability of the virus, the scams and scares they could showcase just then. But, in hindsight, it looks like a massively well-organised global PR work. The matter for propaganda was ready in some clinical labs, in some parts of the world already.

To the world, it seemed to be China's ploy; after having lost its battle for making its currency the world currency, by replacing the U.S. dollar. China has already tasted the success of its hired PR work by making WHO speak for it and creating a big clout in Afro-Asian countries. The outbreak of viral infection in the wet market of Wuhan could be looked at through the same glass. If it was China's plan, it lost to the western pharmaceutical leaders. China's stocks were put on hold, as its trick was slowly being unveiled. China expected a clean implementation as it had already set fear worldwide and was backed by the World Health Organisation (WHO). But instead, it faced a backlash. The Chinese firm, Sinopharm's anti-Covid-19 vaccine was not much accepted, even after China started inoculating its citizens first. The western world returned Covid-19 preventive shipments from China. When China was all set to rule the terrifying world of Covid-19, the smarter western pharmaceutical companies seized the opportunity.

India waited until the third week of March 2020 with great optimism, although the first case of Covid-19 in India was reported on 5th March 2020. But the media wasn't active yet, and soon the fear of how lethal the novel virus would be intimidated the government. In a democratic country, the government is accountable for playing fouls with neglect. The Indian government acted but eventually overacted without any prudence. But the recklessness of their decisions couldn't be questioned by anyone because everyone wanted the authority to act tough and contain the virus's spread. The fear spiralled through media, law, authority, and human seclusion. A novel virus had created a novel situation, and in the absence of a strong code of conduct, the lawmakers ruled. A section of the healthcare business thus took advantage of public fear of having the wanton support of the lawmakers and bureaucrats. The media was used as an ally to instil more fear and promote specific medicines as the only cure.

Soon, the world media was brimming with the news of the catastrophe COVID was creating; virologists, clinical scientists, WHO, Indian and Foreign Governments, as well as medical practitioners, were offering their opinion about the virus.

It was peak summer in India, and April turned out to be the cruellest month. The heat wave was terrible, and the world was strapped indoors under the mandatory lockdown, and the health workers enveloped in PPE kits served the infected. While on one side, India was groping in the dark like other nations, on the other side, it was overwhelmed and irrationally over-cautious. India, unlike other nations, has rich traditional healthcare to boast about. But everything was uncertain at this time and in the haste of testing medicines for hope, our traditional healthcare was overlooked. However, some medical expert's opinions about using home medicine spread like wildfire through social media, and the result was spectacular.

The socio-economic impacts of the pandemic-induced lockdown from 26th March 2020 in India was an emotionally moving period as an exodus of workers from urban centres after their worksites were locked, started walking their way to their hometowns thousands of kilometres across the country, while the other segments of society remained safe indoors. In the absence of transportation and state borders sealed, it was utter chaos these daily wage workers bore at the hands of fear and livelihood. Lockdown made poor people sicker and poorer while the immoral ones became richer. Lawmakers and regulators of healthcare segments went wrong, and behind the pandemic curtain, what went on secretly could be a matter of investigation. But hope was set on nature's equation, that every truth shall be unveiled one day.

The 21st-century Covid-19 pandemic could either be something more than a nature-induced pandemic or created by someone with a massive plan. Bio-warfare, who knows? If not bio-warfare, perhaps a big commercial bet on heavily influencing international bodies and governments of many countries. After World War II, and the tragic collapse of all dictators, no tyrant dared to nurse such a devastating dream of controlling the world, at least by military occupation. But strategically, by bringing the entire world to be controlled by remote control.

Chinese Virologist, Dr. Li-Meng's controversial claim of the novel coronavirus being made in a government-controlled laboratory in Wuhan cannot be put under the carpet. The Americans and the European's fury against China couldn't be termed racial or provincial. China reportedly tried to cover up the epidemic against which WHO was accused of being silent. The U.S. was furious about it and even threatened to defend WHO for its inaction. WHO, which initially claimed that the use of masks was unnecessary, remained a silent spectator when China denied them independent access to Wuhan for an investigation. In the meantime, China ramped up the production of masks and personal protective equipment (PPE), and so did Taiwan. China readied mass production before the world was waking up to the alert. It saw the world was getting ready to cry for its chaos, while it was bracing business and ruling strategies.

While it was only a while ago that China miserably lost a trade war with the United States of America, its game plan to make the Yuan the world's reserve currency failed. Its dream of hegemony was shattered. On the other hand, we also cannot deny the unhappiness of the U.S. with the WHO. The latest developments across the world and many factors circumstantially indicated every suspicion of a conspiracy, with a firm and irrefutable base.

The book deals with the history of pandemics and how human beings are prepared for managing the pandemic. How man-made catastrophes in nature dealt with nasty emperors by triggering invisible elements, and how nasty rulers dealt with their denizens for holding on and expanding their empires.

Medical science, which is supposed to serve sick human beings, has become a tool of business for corporate sharks. And when this business began to thrive, human life was put on a trial neglecting the tribulations of the entire human world, barring the tip of the socio-economic pyramid. Though the virus did not discriminate between rich and poor, our socio-economic status defined the nature of treatment that we receive. In a pandemic situation, our healthcare mechanism explored commercial propositions giving in to vested interests.

No one has, to this date, questioned how the pandemic management plans all over the world failed miserably, in the days when the world started catching a cold and China stopped sneezing. As China knew that Covid-19 was set to storm the world, the Wuhan Institute of Virology filed a patent for the use of Remdesivir in China in the third week of January 2020, after securing approval from the original owner of the drug. If not Ebola, let it be for Covid-19, Remdesivir hence coincidentally found a target. Although it was later found to have serious side effects, and we are all witnesses to the enormous mess-up on decisions proposed by healthcare regulators. The inconsistent talks from scientists on the nature of the virus and too many inconsistent treatment protocols all over the world. These talks continued through the 10th month after the Covid-19 breakout. The way untargeted medicines were used for treating Covid-19 could cause more damage to the health of Covid-19 victims than good. Post-recovery, many people slipped into other health complications as the reactive indications of certain drugs administered to them. Whereas those who could manage recovery through home remedies and traditional medicines haven't reported many complications. The constantly changing treatment protocol and a gradual easing of the treatment framework were suggestive of the medical fraternity's perplexities over the core issues of the epidemic.

The book addresses the role played by India's traditional medicines in supporting the war against the pandemic and why modern medicine is at a loggerhead. Despite encouraging a desirable and discrete integration with it. This part also unravels the medical sector's ruthless business orientation to a painful extent. It is not the virus that troubles the world, but the mad rush to make human beings sick as a customer target. If the pandemic triggered sales of many drugs, the post-pandemic has opened a bigger market for vaccination and post-Covid treatment. The persisting fear would make people inoculate the newborns and take the mandatory doses themselves. Again, it's a larger scope of business than was envisioned.

The book also dwells on our policymaker's miscalculations and where we failed in tackling the pandemic. It is perhaps a human error that contributes to the aggravation of every calamity and the consequent economic disaster. This part underlines the lessons that we must learn in changing the socio-economic atmosphere and how a new world is emerging for a safer and better quality of life after the crisis, even when people binge on their hope for Covid vaccination.

Chapter 3

When the Government Declared Lockdown

In March 2020, optimistic hearts felt the pandemic could be controlled through some early measures. But the lockdown frightened the people and rendered more serious concerns about job loss, social distancing, and making ends meet. For many families, the lockdown came to be a disaster.

Migrant workers landed in uncertainty, and urban highways carried a heart-melting and depriving look of these migrant's exodus.

Initially, many people thought the lockdown would bring effective control over the pandemic within 3 weeks. On the other side, the decision was criticised for being a sudden imposition, as it was done without preparation for meeting eventualities arising out of bringing everything to a sudden halt. Many people were furious about the long-drawn lockdown, which they termed a collective.

Prime Minister Narendra Modi called for a Janata curfew on 22nd March 2020, and the next day evening, he declared a nationwide 21-day lockdown. This caught everyone off guard as they were not at all ready for this turn of events.

Every work was stopped, except the extreme emergency ones. People were stopped from moving out. People abided by the lockdown because of fear; one, the fear of Covid-19, and 2, fear of the ruthless police action if caught outside during a lockdown. The atmosphere was terrifyingly calm, and the blistering heat of the arriving summers made the situation worse.

I assisted people in procuring Ayurvedic medicines, and this was an ongoing endeavour during the lockdown. Not bothering about the infection, effort was put into making the medicines that had to reach people. It was evident that the creation of fear among people was a ploy. The lockdown was only an imprudent and weak defensive measure after all. After making a prudent estimation of how my body and mind worked, I acted accordingly. I used to commute locally daily for more than 40 km, to understand the impact and genesis of the infection.

During my commute, I noticed many people walking tiresomely with a backpack and heavy baggage on their shoulders and head. Some were carrying their children with them, besides other family members. They had no option but to brave the simmering summer heat and walk towards their faraway destination- their hometown.

The lockdown had created 2 sections of people; one section resolutely stayed behind their locked doors, and the other section left for their safer native place without the aid of a transport service. Every worksite closed indefinitely since March 26, the day the devastating lockdown began abruptly. There were no social workers or volunteers on the roadside either to protect these people or support them to reach a safer place, except for the hostile police. These people did every job that was grimy, filthy, and risky. Who worked in raising the city. Today, there was no one when they needed help.

It was a human tragedy, as millions of migrant workers took to the highways in desperation, often walking hundreds or even thousands of kilometres back to their home villages. According to a conservative estimate, this was the largest internal migration in recent human history.

The migrant workers had a misadventure, on which they embarked after they lost their jobs. Without a job, they knew they were unable to sustain their necessities in big cities.

The government paid no heed to this crisis, even as people were dying on the roads and trains. There have been cases where workers walked 1500 kilometres or more to get to the safe confines of their native place, where at least shelter and food could be procured. This was a tragedy of epic proportions.

The irony was these migrant workers who finally returned to their villages were no longer welcome in many cases. In several villages located in the states of Bihar and Jharkhand, for example, villagers had put up barricades and posters at entry points with warnings that migrants must go through a health check before being allowed into the village.

The pandemic has had an extreme impact on domestic migrants in India, with the poor and marginalised bearing the brunt of the crisis. Migrants died from starvation, exhaustion, road and rail accidents, police brutality, and denial of timely medical care.

Their sweat-drenched bodies did not even have water to drink or refill as all shops were shut, roadside water taps were closed, and no humans were offering any service. They had to fend for themselves and take their families safely back to their hometown. The state transport was shut, the cross-state borders were closed and in all this, they just kept walking with just one quest of reaching their hometown, a safe abode. They were unafraid of Covid, but they were more afraid of spending days without earning a living.

These workers looked deeply dejected, tortured, and on their faces reflected a loss of every hope. Political rivals of the government had a field day, and journalists wrote story after story about them, but nothing was done to attract help.

However, later it was proved, migrant's decision to return home at the very moment their worksite was shut was a safe decision. The cities where the migrant labourers were based later saw a massive spread of infection that would have made their life more chaotic, especially in the context of the treatment cost and sustaining without work and salary. Their decision was right as they could move to their safer native village to at least do farming.

As Covid-19 caseloads continued to rise in big cities, India's rural villages were much safer. People in rural areas had no fear and hardly bothered to wear a mask, as they felt completely safe in their zones. The migrating labourers, who felt safer at their native place, became financially more comfortable and optimistic. At least half of them wouldn't like to return to cities. By the end of 6 months after the lockdown, factories and construction sites that used to depend on migrant labours were yet to resume their full-fledged commercial operations.

The suddenly imposed lockdown was termed as a collective miscalculation and unjustifiably hasty decision after people understood and experienced its unsaid drawbacks. The sudden lockdown was more severe and testing than an unpredicted natural calamity. It hit people mentally.

In factories, work remained half-done and in some cases, factory machines couldn't stop all of a sudden. Long haulage trailers carrying goods from the factory to market could not be halted mid-way. In India, we were just around the financial year-end, and organisations were preparing for rigorous audits and sales closures. Some people were even deciding where to spend their summers, in their hometown or on vacation, and the lockdown was suddenly imposed out of the blue.

Initially, I thought it was a mistake of India alone. Like India, most countries had taken such decisions partly or fully. In a democracy, rulers are generally afraid of public outcry and accountability over all mishaps caused by legislative missteps. Middle and low-income classes lost all hope and did not know what awaited them.

Thousands of people lost their jobs in just 3 months as the lockdown began. In small companies, retrenchment was as high as three-fourths. Though the Prime Minister had announced not to fire anyone from their job and not to cut salaries, small companies could only do what they found necessary. They did not have funds to sustain or bear salaries. For project works, the government issued Force Majeure. Even public sector enterprise contractors fired their subcontractors, landing them in severe financial crises and irreparable losses. The government had announced an arrangement for liberal bank loans. Businesses were already facing the order not to retrench employees and had to bear their salaries without making any profit. And, these loans were further death traps, and this is what every business thought in the uncertain Covid scenario.

The businesses, especially small ones, were kept under pressure. Notices from tax departments, various types of penal charges, and inflated utility bills never stopped despite the pandemic, and it further broke their already broken back. Businesses felt orphaned. Public servants too remained oblivious to the pains of businesses and their struggles unless there were strict special orders from the government. None came forward to enlighten them about the risk they should be ready to deal with.

Urbanites, who were in deeper trouble, were disappointed over the uncalculated and hasty decision of a long lockdown. Every sensible person would have wished the government to make an elaborate preparation and asked people to be ready for a lockdown at least a week before so that each citizen could have taken their position and planned. By strictly directing people to maintain social distancing, the government could have given everyone a chance to settle down at a place of their choice. Before resorting to such a war-time-like decision, the government should have let people make necessary arrangements to sustain. The sudden lockdown announcement crippled the healthcare system also since the healthcare providers didn't have time to prepare for any eventuality.

The government should have also asked all foreigners to leave the country and suspended all international flights subsequently since January for foreign nationals. Homecoming Indians could have been made to live in quarantine and tested for their health condition. Lockdown was a mismanaged chaos, and it changed the entire world not only by contracting the economy but inducing a change in the socio-economic equation.

While those without a voice suffered worse, those who were ineligible for any government hand-out got away with it, despite enough systems to monitor the foul play. The rural countryside that led to a reverse flow of migrants in the cities was the next big challenge. But nothing of that happened. Rural India was able to accept its children back into its womb, and that too without much ado.

Chapter 4

Fear and Anxiety

Fear is a state of mind emerging from guessing or sensing danger in any form, physical or mental. Fear that makes one move cautiously, in a way, protects him or her from vulnerability awaiting. Every creature on the planet carries this nature. It is a universal emotion that every creature is endowed with. It haunts every living being.

Fear is an instinctive, powerful, and primitive feeling that has existed ever since humans originated. Every creature on the planet is inherently driven by fear. It is a natural phenomenon. It is a feeling that animals have in the presence of a predator or in being alert, but we humans suffer from fear.

Fear has reformed in different ways in humans over the course of their brain development. While fear was just physical in the primitive human, today it has extended physically, socially, monetarily, psychologically, and emotionally. Humans are fearful of their future, and in doing so they are losing their present. Because this is one overgrown instinctive feeling rendered by nature, only for a safe and secure existence.

A person who does financially well is always fearful of losing his or her possessions. They are bothered about things that cannot be bought with money. On the other hand, someone who is struggling financially yearns for money. Some fear being dominated by power, some by virtue. We all have some fear or the other. Even a goon, who terrifies all the people around him, has a constant fear of getting murdered by his enemies or being caught by the authorities. And that's the circle of life and fear.

Fear generates unexplainable mental troubles for humans. If a person is suspected of cancer and is advised to do further investigations by a doctor, they get more worried and feel the pain of the disease already, which until then, they might not have suffered. Even if they have only a 50% chance of turning out positive for malignancy, they are already afraid of impending disaster that might not even be true. Instead of garnering hope and confidence, fear completely conquers.

Death anxiety, also known as thanatophobia, is anxiety produced by thoughts of one's death (fear of death).

A heart attack is a result of people's lifestyle. Due to half-knowledge, any simple or severe pain on the left side of the body frightens us and makes us run with fear and anxiety to the nearest doctor. Gastritis and muscle pain also have identical symptoms. Doctor's of Modern Medicine can classify the difference and diagnose correctly.

When a person feels sick, if they control their mind to feel relaxed or fit, it will aid a lot in fighting and overcoming the sickness. We have seen many examples of people who have conquered physical ailments with the power of a strong mentality.

Fear works both defensively and offensively. If fear nudges us to stay distracted from possible hazards, fear acts as a defensive factor too. On the other hand, sometimes fear dissipates a positive spirit, therefore leading to a negative or unwanted outcome.

Let's imagine that you were having food continuously from a restaurant until last week. Suddenly one day, you came to know that the restaurant was raided by the food quality department and found out that they were serving stale food for a long time. What would happen to you on hearing this? Your mind takes over, and now you may feel nausea, stomachache, or even vomiting at the thought of the stale food you had. Although it didn't cause any damage to you at that time. But why is it happening now? It's human psychology. If you say to your mind, the body will prepare for it, that is the truth. There is a beautiful anecdote representing this.

A group of scientists conducted a study about the psychology of human minds on a prisoner sentenced to death. As part of the experiment, they told him that his death verdict will be execution by a cobra bite. Now, panic attacks are already thought in the mind of the prisoner about being bitten by a cobra.

As a part of the experiment, on the day of the execution, he was made to sit on a chair, and a cobra was brought in front of him. He was then blindfolded, and the authorities pricked him with a pin. The unexpected part is, he died of the prick! How was this possible? It is the strength of the mind to lead the body to do anything it strongly and adamantly believes in.

Now let's correlate this psychology to the Covid-19 situation. Since the onset of the pandemic, a morbid and panic situation was plotted in the name of the coronavirus, through various media outfits. The alerts, unstable expert comments, videos of darting ambulances, piling dead bodies, and many horrible scenes were visually scary and made people fear. Instead, people should have been given a morale boost that they shouldn't be afraid of the viral infection.

Did you during the pandemic hear such a piece of advice from anyone seriously? No! All we heard were symptoms, and death counts. No one took the effort of building the confidence that was required more than any medicine. Extreme fear or terror about a disease changes the chemistry of the body. The outburst of certain alert hormones peaks in the human body which makes us think that we are sick. More than a viral Covid infection, the ailment was mental instability. Any small infection or fever was imagined by the mind as Covid, in such a scenario.

And then on being hospitalised, the terror increased alarmingly. As the doctor evaluated, and the patients nodded to all the symptoms, their mind was pacing ahead making them feel sick, and soon the diagnosis confirmed their fear.

Further, the feeling of being isolated from everyone shattered all the remaining confidence, making the patient overly insecure. The Covid-19 pandemic was testing patients and family members from fear to the funeral. And if someone survived all this ordeal, then they were back home with unexpected complications.

Corona was ruling over the minds more than it existed. It was an endeavour to remain out of all the negative news yet remain informed. The coronavirus pandemic dominated everyone's thoughts through every newspaper's front page stories about the virus; radio and TV programmes had constant coverage of the latest death tolls; and depending on who you follow, social media platforms were filled with frightening statistics, practical advice, or shallow humour. We rarely face such a widespread threat to our health, and it's natural to feel worried or anxious in these circumstances.

As social animals, humans have evolved to live in large groups, and our behavioural immune system has modified our interactions with others to minimise the spread of disease, by instinctively practicing social distancing.

The combination of grieving the loss of a loved one with the added stress of the COVID-19 pandemic can be unbearable for some. Social distancing, 'stay-at-home orders,' and limits on the size of in-person gatherings have forced changes to the way friends and family can gather and grieve, including holding traditional funeral services, regardless of COVID-19 deaths. However, as difficult as these preventive measures may be, they are crucial in slowing down the spread of COVID-19.

Fear, as we see, ruled us all during the COVID-19 scenario, and it has in turn been an ally to the medical and healthcare industry. Modern medicine is one of the best examples of this. The fear of people determines the prospects of certain industries. Ethics seem to have dissipated barring certain cases. Life, the most precious thing for any living being, is risked for materialistic needs and greediness. As humans, when we land in trouble, we understand the importance of life, and we panic to save it. Other living things protect their life as a part of their everyday life. For humans, our life has many priorities before good health, and it's time we humans understood that and live a fruitful life as long as we are alive.

Adolf Jest

Hundreds of years ago, Dr. Adolf Jest wrote a book, 'The Return to Nature.' In his book, he explained the power of mental health in curing illness. He was a physician and was fed up with inorganic drug administration in patients. He was in search of an alternative system. Once when he was treating a family who got infected with flu, the man of the house refused to take the drugs as they couldn't afford treatment for everyone. He stayed outside the house and let others take the treatment. The doctor observed later that he recovered perfectly along with others, despite having no medicines.

Dr. Adolf asked the man, "What did he do?" He simply said that he did nothing but stay in the open air due to less space inside the house and didn't have much food due to the sickness. Most importantly, he had ample rest. The doctor concluded, "Rest, fasting, and fresh air were the reasons behind his fast recovery." Then he started giving food grains and water as medicines to his patients without their knowledge. People started recovering. It was the mind that considered food grains and water as medicines. The perception worked against the disease.

Reiki

Reiki healing therapy originated in Japan in the late 1800s involving the transfer of universal energy through the practitioner's palm to their patient. Although it is hard to prove the effectiveness of Reiki on grounds of modern science, where documentation is the only substantial support, thousands of people find relief and recovery through the Reiki system. It ultimately heals the mind. Even if the practitioner and the patients are far away physically, they can communicate well, and the session works for the people.

Reiki works if the person is willing to accept it and trusts in the process. So, for major problems where the mind is the matter, a solution lies in our psychological approach. Many streams of medicine have evolved over the years. Modern medicine is the only one among them that has been fostered through business opportunities. A healthcare stream with a business dimension is a contradiction. But we accepted it as a part of life. While considering this the most popular stream of medicine. We shouldn't believe that other streams are unworkable. Advocates of the modern medical system don't support any indigenous system, pointing at the lack of documentation and pieces of evidence. That is not the correct perception. A change is needed, and an integrated system will serve us better.

Importance of life

Now we understand the importance of oxygen very well. Without it, we can't survive. Oxygen works like an elixir of life. Severely infected COVID-19 patients suffered oxygen deficiency, which was a major concern. But once we are beyond these testing experiences, we forget the importance of these experiences and their impact on us.

Once we return to our comfortable and cosy life, we forget the pain and misery. We think living in the modern world with a modern lifestyle is called civilised. But if we ponder, we get to know where we belong. We are the latest of the homos grappling with unnatural life. We were once thinking instinctively, learning from experiences, and responding logically.

Our body is the most spectacular machine ever. If it is infected, it has an auto system to repair itself. Our conscious mind and instinctive actions should work on the repair mechanism the body has. But we are not doing it. Do you know the best way to prevent any disease, including Corona? It's a healthy lifestyle and a confident mind. In Ayurvedic texts, the first thing explained is, your body is the Maha Vaidya, which was not there before your birth. That implies your immunity and the power of the body to protect you from any ailment. During a simple fever also, we pop up pills instead of staying back and resting by allowing the body to do its work. No logical thinking at all! These are all results of the inorganic life in which we are living. And fear plays its role.

Chapter 5

Modern Medicine Before Medicine is Modernised

> "Physician must convert or insert wisdom into medicine, and medicine to wisdom." – Hippocrates

Though Hippocrates, who lived in the 5th century, was known as the father of modern medicine. Even the oath that new physicians take today asks to swear upon several healing gods, to uphold a number of professional ethical standards. Ironically, no modern medicine that is currently in use has its origin more than 2 centuries ago leaving the Hippocrates era. Many medicines, which were introduced to target the pain of human beings, could only add more pain. Drug regulators in many countries had later withdrawn the approval of such medicines.

The Government of India has a list of more than 440 drugs that are prohibited for manufacture and sale. At the top of the anti-inflammatory list is pyrazolone with analgesic, anti-inflammatory, and antipyretic properties, which was found to have the risk of agranulocytosis. This medicine was synthesised by Friedrich Stolz, a German chemist, who was the first person to artificially synthesise adrenaline along with another German chemist, Ludwig Knorr. Most of the medicines, which are now banned, were in use for many decades before they were declared lethal.

Hippocrates used only plant-based medicine harnessing the strength of nature and wisdom, which were not different from Ayurveda in India. Hippocrates died at the age of 104.

The ancient Indian physician and surgeon, Sushruta, who was known as the father of surgery, lived much before Hippocrates. Ancient scholars, without the luxury of supercomputers and other technical support, could understand the inside of the human body. Both Charaka and Shushruta treated patients and used painkillers from plants in their treatments. Although it was not after any clinical trial, Hippocrates treated plague victims in Athens. His quote, "Physician must convert or insert wisdom into medicine and the medicine to wisdom," seems so much to ponder on. Ayurveda, which was popular before the era of Hippocrates, was also the proponent of wisdom.

In previous centuries, no diseases other than bacterial and viral infections were known to have killed human beings, and we still see these as causes of death today. Maybe medical history hasn't recorded anything like death from other causes such as genetic disorders. We see this from alarming instances of sickness among people who recovered from COVID-19 with the support of modern medicines. That is going to be a big challenge. Patients were helpless as their freedom was curtailed under the frame of government protocol and the regime of the Epidemic Act. It practically brought in a prohibition on the traditional way of treatment.

Today, with modern medicine, after all drug trials and rigorous approval mechanisms, infection is used to treat other illnesses.

The Delta variant has been more successful than any other form of COVID, causing countries with stringent border controls like Australia and China to close their borders. Its been the deadliest form of COVID for most of this year, with more than 3.5 million people have died from the virus.

Every year, 5.2 million medical errors occur in India according to a study by Harvard. Medical errors in hospitals kill more people each year than motor vehicle wrecks, breast cancer, and AIDS combined. Among the several factors that can contribute to medical errors, the most commonly identified ones are miscommunication and inadequate information exchange.

The COVID-19 pandemic has increased the rate of medical errors and is a leading cause of harm and death globally. Before the pandemic, medical errors were the third leading cause of death in the U.S., but the pandemic quickly surpassed that. However, medical errors are still a silent killer that doesn't get much media attention, thus keeping people clueless.

A major challenge during COVID-19 was the absence of any single approved drug that could have a significant effect on the virus with few or no side effects. According to available evidence, many anti-viral and anti-inflammatory drugs were used to treat patients without knowledge of the consequences. Additionally, the patient's immune response played a pivotal role in the development of COVID-19, so managing anxiety, delirium, and agitation became an added situation to be encountered.

Medication misadventure includes any iatrogenic incidents associated with a medical examination or adverse drug events (ADE's), medication errors (MEs), or adverse drug reactions (ADRs).

The United States National Coordinating Council for Medication Error Reporting and Prevention (NCC-MERP) defines Medical

Error as 'Any preventable event that may cause or lead to inappropriate medication use or harm patients while the medication is in the control of the healthcare professional (HCP's), patient, or consumer.'

Given the rampant and often unproven drug usage during COVID-19, it is crucial that we evaluate the impact of these medications on misadventures such as MEs (medication errors) and ADRs (adverse drug reactions).

The month of October 2020 was a good one for Gilead Sciences, the anti-viral drug manufacturer based in Foster City, California. On October 8th, the company signed an agreement to supply the European Union with its drug Remdesivir as a treatment for COVID-19—a deal that could be worth more than $1 billion. Two weeks later, on October 22nd, the U.S. Food and Drug Administration (FDA) approved Remdesivir for use against the pandemic coronavirus SARS-CoV-2 in the United States—the first drug to receive that status.

The decisions of the European Union and the United States have set the stage for Gilead's drug to enter 2 markets that were struggling with increasing COVID-19 cases. However, these decisions left scientists scratching their heads, as the clinical trials for Remdesivir have raised many questions about its effectiveness over the past 6 months.

The most recent trial, conducted by the World Health Organisation, was published on October 15th, 2020, and showed that Remdesivir does not reduce mortality rates or the recovery time for COVID-19 patients. This news came as a blow to Gilead and has left many scientists wondering if the drug is worth pursuing.

But amidst all this, the masses were subjected to the remdesivir drug. Even back in India, the drug was highly sought and attracted a whopping black market price amidst controversies.

In another shocking revelation, French virologist and Nobel Prize winner Luc Montagnier called mass vaccination against the coronavirus during the pandemic 'unthinkable' and a historical blunder that is 'creating the variants' and leading to deaths from the disease.

"A scientific error as well as a medical error. It is an unacceptable mistake," he said. "The history books will show that because it is the vaccination that is creating the variants. Many epidemiologists know it and are silent about the problem known as an antibody-dependent enhancement. It is the antibodies produced by the virus that enable an infection to become stronger, while variants of viruses can occur naturally."

Chapter 6

The Virus Mystery and Overzealous Actions

Some scientists with ulterior motives can regenerate viruses to devastate the human race. The Hiroshima and Nagasaki bombings were the result of such extraordinary brain works. In the history of mankind, there are plenty of examples of mass killings to dominate the world with conventional weapons. The new world dictators and rulers with a desire to control the world may doubt their chance of winning a war with conventional weapons to dominate the world. But there are other powerful avenues, and none can rule out a bio-weapon delivery in the form of a virus. The concerns of capitalist interests also loom large.

According to scientists, a virus is only a lifeless particle, which acquires some power with spiked protein when it enters the cellular system. Outside the human body, the virus neither has a chance to multiply nor invade the place it has occupied.

In fact, a virus has no life outside the cellular system. In the same way, we cannot live outside the atmosphere. Quite astonishing, right? That is what our scientists say unanimously. As human beings, can we ever be dormant outside and active inside some cell? The plain answer is 'No.' The size is a matter, as nature has made us so. The same nature has set a mystery for the communicable particle, Virus - a Latin word meaning liquid poison. In Middle English, it means poisonous secretion. But is this a poison that can kill human beings? Scientists say the poisonous particle called the virus has a life of only 14 days within the human body. If all the viruses could kill human beings within 14 days, the human race would have been extinct from the planet long ago. But great nature has set a balanced ecosystem for every living being, including microbes.

For this reason, most people who are infected by this 'poison' survive through a nature-endowed resistance called immunity. As it is generally said, nature has given all living beings an inbuilt defensive system to fight against external bodies and kill them within. Viral infection has a history of over 80 million years. Because of this, no human intervention can eradicate any kind of virus. The presence of the virus only demands a highly immunised system to control it, and that is a natural system. At the same time, the virus particle will continue to come up with different pathogenicity, and that is unstoppable. Vaccination may only help the medical fraternity to stop calling another round of infection as Covid-19.

Viral infections will keep surfacing and will be known by different names. Vaccination cannot rule out a revisit of a pandemic. Another virus, another pandemic, another vaccine—the process will be infinite. The best way, perhaps the only way to resist all future worries, is to take care of one's immune system, which would enable resisting the virus.

We have forgotten this fundamental factor and started worrying about a virus that couldn't even be seen with an ordinary microscope. Yet, when the virus unleashed its attack, medical science remained helpless. The source of virus emergence, whether it is by default of nature or by human creation, is still a question. Whatever the source, the novel coronavirus tested modern medical science. Ironically, medical science should have tested the virus to understand its pathogenic character. The virus overran all labs, defeating the scientist's endeavour to understand it, but for an ultimate claim to victory by modern medical science for having saved 96 per cent of the virus victims.

Many of the recoveries were by chance. The mortality was the result of miscalculation and wrong judgement of the medical fraternity. On earth, viruses and bacteria have billions of years-long histories. Questions like which country was infected first and how many people died of viral and bacterial infections couldn't be answered by anyone, thanks to the hidden creation of nature.

According to some information, the coronavirus was first discovered in the 1930s when an acute respiratory infection of domesticated chickens was shown to be caused by the infectious bronchitis virus. In human beings, the virus was said to have been discovered in the 1960s. In the last 6 decades, scientists have been on a vigorous search. In this context, is it sensible to call the virus novel?

If we continue to argue about the novelty of the virus and resolutely say that the new virus infection, called Covid-19, is novel, then it is an indirect admission of our ignorance about the power of nature and human research of all these decades. What is supposed to be called novel is the engineered lab-borne microorganism made by some savages with a scientific brain. Coronavirus and too many other viruses reside in every living being and in the environment.

Since the day it was found in laboratories, it is considered to be pathogenic in our bodies. We termed it novel, fatal, dangerous, and so on. Human being's natural interaction with other living organisms is not new.

The co-existence of a virus with the human world is unavoidable. A virus is not fully eradicable. When the inevitability of nature is taken for analysis, and suspicious ones are separated, our scientists found something to call enemies of human beings. The enemy target then evolved into new medical theories. Then we employed modern science to suppress it and devastate the existence of particular pathogens. Eventually, antibiotics were created to kill them. However, creation is infinite. When one virus is eradicated, another unstoppably emerges and lives longer.

In 1928, the Scottish Physician, Alexander Fleming discovered penicillin. It took more than a decade to introduce it for any treatment, which was said to be a turning point in the history of medical science. Fleming himself admitted that his discovery was accidental. He did not know the significance. The scientific world too did not understand Fleming's discovery. Later, it led to a path-breaking solution for infections. Years passed, and millions had been inoculated with penicillin. Subsequently, across the globe, labs have worked on measures to repair the damage it inflicted on human beings.

We also find research as another business opportunity. As I have said in my other book, 'By Heart,' research is a bigger damage, built on an existing and another big damage to derive a desirable result.

As we are afraid of the notorious Covid-19 or any other virus or bacteria, we need to understand the fact that it is only because of our undesirable practice. The undesirable practice leads to self-destruction either through a pandemic or through some natural calamities. We know there are many places on the planet that human brains cannot reach easily, maybe because of restrictions, fear, or adverse conditions. The virus is a creation of nature either by default or by culturing at research laboratories. In this context, who is the right person to say what its character is? Many scientists have varying opinions. The experts have a different opinion, and it is authentic. With differing news, people are confused every time a new version of the argument comes up.

Even when the truth is hardly ascertained, the findings of the so-called scientists become the unquestionable conclusion. We are talking and making tall claims. When we see bats hanging down a tree, it is not a concern for anyone. But when we think to climb up and catch one to explore, study, or eat, set aside the alert that they may be dangerous, it is an unnatural activity. That creates chaos, which may be normal for those who deal with such activities routinely.

Modern life science has killed more people, often groping in the dark as it couldn't make a stable profile of the worst pandemic of 2 centuries, despite many boastful achievements in its stride. It failed in developing targeted drugs, and a final solution was found in vaccination. Vaccination only means immunisation, which nature has given to every human being. All the traditional medicines target only this aspect. While vaccination is externally inducing drugs to immune, to be ready to fight, natural immunity keeps the human body naturally fit for fighting the virus.

Building immunity within the body is the core of the Ayurvedic treatment tradition. Ever since the Covid-19 pandemic alert was sent out, scholarly Ayurvedic doctors have told this truth, which the larger medical world refused to believe. While vaccination prevents the possibility of an infection, Ayurveda treats the patient and keeps him or her ready to fight future infection. According to an Ayurvedic doctor signs and symptoms similar to Covid-19 manifestations have been observed in many disease contexts also.

In many instances, complications of fever as sudden onset led to unstable vitals also. But all those manifestations are not Covid-19. In the Ayurvedic perspective, communicable diseases are termed

Sankramika Rogas. Whereas immunity can be interpreted as *belam* or *vyadhikshamathwam* (Acharya Sushruta). In Ayurvedic contexts, the resistance against the disease has been narrated as the strength of the body to disable pathogenesis or the immune response of the body not to create favourable endogenic reactions.

Though the mortality rate is not so high, there is a big space for fear. Those who recovered from the infection after excessive exposure to modern medicines report life-threatening side effects. Further treatment based on reports of biomarkers further complicates their illness. The recovery is only a feeling of temporary tranquillisation. The medicines hinder the natural immunity of the human body. While the high dosages discount the immunity level, excessive medicines weaken the body, perhaps for a longer period.

Chapter 7

Death By Virus and Bacteria

Coronavirus was invisible to the naked eye yet powerful for medical science to comprehend. While boasting of making headway, medical science failed to overcome the so-called killer virus. WHO declared the Coronavirus as a large family of viruses that cause illnesses ranging from the common cold to SARS-CoV and MERS-CoV.

Be it mild, moderate, or severe, the Corona Virus shook the entire world.

The world knew about Covid-19 after China reported a rare type of pneumonia. But it is referred to in classic medical books in Greece and much before it, in Indian Ayurveda too.

The virus is a particle, inactive outside and dominantly active inside a cellular system. Nature is known to have created non-living forms before setting the mysterious chemistry of organic compounds that acted and reacted through long processes. It all happened billions of years ago, and so did the evolution of life. The formation of RNA and DNA happened in its wake. Scientists trampled long roads to find the origin of energies that initiated evolution but did not have been in much luck.

Viruses and bacteria were also created by nature in the same format, yet surprisingly with no change over billions of years. Hence, eradication of viruses and bacteria, as creations of nature, is not easy. One can only be accepting and modulating with what nature desires. Nature has its ways to educate us on what is right and wrong. The denial of the order of nature has always been ruthlessly compensated for, and this we would know as we read every pandemic story that human history has seen so far.

While scientists could locate the invisible virus through an extraordinary microscope, medical science, despite all boasting about making much headway, failed to eradicate it with a drug.

The virus becomes inactive only by the natural immunity created within the human body and albeit it killed several hundred thousand people living in the most advanced countries. How is that possible? The entire world was terrified and halted on its toes searching in panic for a quick solution. No one knew how many more human lives were to be sacrificed in the name of the pandemic. All the clinical scientists worldwide were burning the midnight oil in search of a solution. On the other hand, some had hired big brains and were waiting anxiously to find a solution and make a business fortune out of it.

As the initial stories of viral infection devastating Wuhan, China occurred in January 2020, neglecting similar reports in the previous month, it was obvious that this is the strategy of someone, who was simultaneously getting ready with an antidote to this virus. In a couple of months, the virus crossed the Atlantic through its eastern exit over to California in the U.S. and the Mediterranean over to Italy. Both these countries would then be the worst sufferers of the pandemic. The economic capital of the world, New York had been in chaos with dead bodies piling up for last rites. Fifteen months later we saw the same scenario in some Indian states.

Rich and poor countries have arsenals built over trillions of dollars. They were all powerless to defeat the virus, further considered as a man-made killer that rebelled out of the lab. However, the virus travelled around the world silently with travellers by transmitting even in the world's much-talked-about safest zones.

The disease management capability of the superior developed economies in the world, which used to indulge in dictating standards for developing countries like India was put to test. The novel coronavirus hit millions with several hundred thousand mortalities even in boastfully developed countries like the U.S. and almost every European country. Italy, the birthplace of the Renaissance, was the worst hit with maximum coronavirus fatalities. The 21st century was facing the challenge of bracing up for a battle against the pandemic that rattled the world in a matter of days.

In world history, wars, political conflicts, and natural calamities might not have killed so many people as viruses and bacteria have until the last century. Although there is no definite count of the number of deaths by viruses and bacteria, tentatively over a billion people have been killed until the fag-end of the 20th century.

The plague was the most notorious in the bacterium infection category acquired through direct contact with infected animals, unlike the novel coronavirus that spreads rapidly through human-to-human transmission. While the plague attacks made many empires, including the most powerful Roman and Greek empires fall, historians and medical scientists lost count of the number of deaths by tuberculosis caused by mycobacterium since the evolution of the human species. Big armies lost their battle against bacterial infection until the saviour ammunition called antibiotics was developed in the 20th century. Even with the discovery of antibiotics, the human kingdom hasn't been protected from virus and bacteria-driven diseases. With the evolution of human beings, everything around them also evolves; so do viruses and bacteria. A great number of human resources also had been spent on studies, developments, and trials, and the amount of wealth deployed in this process was also not ascertainable. While the plague is almost eradicated barring some nonfatal incidents in the U.S. and China, tuberculosis hasn't yet stopped killing people in Africa. In India, it is still killing an average of 4 lakh people a year, despite a strong treatment protocol in place. In highly impoverished African countries, the rate may be much higher. Africa reports a quarter of the world's tuberculosis deaths.

In the fourteenth century's 'Black Death,' over 400 million people died of the plague in Europe alone. The infection didn't spare knights and soldiers, cardinals and scientists, virologists, and microbiologists. The most treacherous tyrants like King John, who murdered the legitimate inheritor of the crown, Prince Arthur, and his nephew, were defeated by dysentery caused by parasites in the gut. Ten centuries before him, Roman emperor Lucius Verus had died of the plague.

In the last 15 years, according to a report by the WHO, 15.2 million deaths out of the total 56.9 million deaths recorded worldwide in 2016 were caused neither by viruses nor by bacteria but by ischaemic heart disease and stroke. This is the single biggest killer of human beings.

Going by the WHO report, the second biggest killer also hasn't been any virus or bacteria, but chronic obstructive pulmonary disorder. Half a century ago, a U.S. Surgeon General quoted, "The time has come to close the book on infectious disease. We have wiped out infection in the United States." Then came a rally of infections, which opened newer space for medical science. I call it a business with a very powerful influence because of its approach. Then came stories on Human Immunodeficiency Virus (HIV-1) causing Acquired Immunodeficiency Syndrome (AIDS) first in the United States of America. Its roots were traced in Cameroon in Africa transmitted from chimpanzees. But the genomic fusion in the course of evolution helped new world monkeys to resist the virus.

After spreading fear about HIV around the world, another African origin called Severe Acute Respiratory Syndrome (SARS) broke out. Ebola, which has a high mortality rate of over 50 per cent, emerged in the West African country of Sudan in 1976. In Sudan, the mortality rate of Ebola was as high as over two-thirds of the infected. It is a part of retroviruses, which killed more than the population of Canada since the 1980s. The Hepatitis C virus was discovered, and then came the strike of an avian flu pandemic. All these impacts were limited, though the dangers still loom.

But none of the infectious viruses generated so big a commotion and fear around the world as Covid-19 did.

A global lockdown for months made the world come to a halt, negating the gains of decades. It still looms and threatens with its aftereffects. Brisk activities in research labs went on while one report was negated by another, and so many countries and companies were on the track of research, racing to reach the finishing point - a vaccine. The world that was looming in shock took some relief from the positive news and panicked over negative ones. Nevertheless, the confusion of the medical world continues with contradictions after contradictions. The policing of all medical and healthcare regulators showed everything was not alright.

A world-famous vaccine scientist and virologist, of Indian African origin, Gita Ramjee died of a novel coronavirus infection in the early stage of the pandemic. BBC broadcasted news that 50 priests around the world died of Corona by the time India entered the second day of the lockdown.

Virus and bacterial infections have killed several hundred thousand people living in the most advanced countries. The virus has killed many celebrities, super-rich men, politicians, ordinary health workers, and police officers alike. The entire world was terrified and halted on its toes, searching in panic for a quick solution and the world economy was bleeding. Incidentally, poor countries remained relatively safe. No one knows how many human lives the pandemic robbed away. And the aftereffects of the Covid-19 pandemic are yet to be seen.

By the end of November 2020, there were more than 170 vaccines at various stages of development and trials. Three were at an advanced stage of trials and 4 were at a pre-clinical stage. By early December, Europe, America, and Asian countries like India were preparing for supplying the first batch. By the end of December 2020, regulators in various countries approved emergency use. The countries like the U.S., UK, Israel, Russia, and China began inoculating the jab. India started the supply on 16th January 2021. By that time, Israel claimed to have inoculated over 10 per cent of its total 8.6 million people. Soon it reported 6.6 per cent of the total number of people who took the jab, tested positive. The people who tested positive included those who took the second dose. Efficacy of the vaccine remained questionable, and many people doubted its effectiveness. Reports of post-inoculation positive test cases further perplexed the people. Some were even afraid of taking the vaccine. Notwithstanding, massive negative propaganda about the vaccine confused people, vaccine makers, and the government. The Indian government came out with a strict warning and ordered strict penal action against any anti-vaccine talks.

Chapter 8

Natural Birth and Unnatural Death

Disease, wars, skirmishes of all kinds, intentional peacetime violence called terrorism, political carnage, natural calamities, or reaction to medicines which were developed for the treatment of some diseases killed countless people. All these circumstances are man-made. In all these, incidentally, there was a direct and indirect role of science. Of course, otherwise, death happens only because of disorders caused either by a disease, an accident or self-inflicted damage such as suicide.

Death is unstoppable even by science or by nature. The vaccines, developed by a large number of companies, will not prevent death but may offer some respite from some infections. Some of the latest vaccines attracted a big question on their efficacy, thus leading to a distrust in public on the overall vaccines.

While human beings toil hard to make life better and more comfortable through science, technology, and brainpower, inadvertently, we are using all these to kill more human beings. Modern states spend trillions to develop weapons of mass destruction in the name of defensive systems. Birth is a natural process, as death is. Both will continue as the order of nature. Death is preventable only by preventing birth, but not by vaccination or remedies of any drug. Drugs can stop birth, as the birth rate can be controlled. But human beings cannot be ruthless to their race by using science and technology to eradicate birth.

Since we have become civilised, we have begun documenting birth and death. This arithmetic process is not very old. Earlier, accounts of birth and death were only estimations and assumptions of historians and archaeologists. Modern technology has enabled us to keep records of birth and death more easily and efficiently. Still, there are many unanswered questions that we try answering with our whims and information that we gather from history, created by historians mostly with self-interests.

Vishwanath Chaudhary, chief cremator in Varanasi, expresses the weight of his profession as the ancient city of Varanasi sees a never-ending flow of Hindus coming to be cremated on the banks of the sacred Ganges river. Hindus believe that by being cremated in Varanasi, their souls will be able to complete their journey to heaven and be released from the cycle of birth and death.

Vishwanath Chaudhary, 39, is the raja, or king, of the Dom caste in Varanasi. "The Dom caste has worked at Varanasi's cremation grounds for generations, and with the recent surge in the number of bodies arriving daily - now up to 100 compared to last year's 15 - the searing heat and leaping flames have become unbearable," he says.

"Our family has been involved in managing crematoriums for generations, and we've never seen anything like this," Chaudhary said. "The situation is horrific - last year was nothing compared to what we're seeing now. At times like this, it's easy to lose sight of humanity."

"The onslaught of bodies has sparked a shortage of wood for the pyres, with vendors raising prices significantly."

If we ask who killed more human beings, I don't think anyone can give a correct answer. Was it science? Science has a direct or indirect stake in all the killing. No one çan exactly count the number of deaths by each reason, though unverifiable estimations may be available.

Death is unstoppable even by science or by nature. So, let's not question it. It is the rule of nature that anything naturally made gives a sustainable result, unlike inorganically made things. Many countries, big and small, have spent a staggering amount buying weapons in the name of defence and tackling the issue of terrorism.

World War I (WW1) was triggered by a 19-year-old Serbian teenager with the assassination of Archduke Franz Ferdinand of Austria and his wife Sophie. Gavrilo Princip, the killer of the couple, felt deeply hurt by the annexation of his country by Austria. The devastating conflict that began exactly a month after the assassination lasted 4 years. But the fundamental reason for the war was uncompromising nationalism, unrealistic egoism, and complex defence treaties between an assorted set of 2 continents, mostly in Europe and to a limited extent in Asia.

World War II (WW II) was the result of an overestimation and miscalculation of the leading military powers about their strengths and vengeance. They had dreamt of ruling the entire world and killing everyone whom they hated. They hadn't dreamt of a colony but the entire earth as their empire. They had misused their powers, misread human capabilities, and shown the hidden barbarism of the human mind.

In both wars, the most powerful forces had to bite the dust. All calculations had gone haywire. Though there wasn't an exact count of death in World War 1, the figure was seen as roughly around 16 million people. But the influenza epidemic killed 50 million people in 1918. Most of the deaths happened within hours of showing the first symptoms. Young ones who naturally showed better resilience to infections also fell. A quarter of the U.S. population fell to the infection.

Of course, death happens only because of disorders caused either by various diseases, including misjudgment of doctors, drug reaction, an accident, or self-inflicted damage that is suicide. It is difficult to call death unnatural as everyone faces its reality. Still, we call death by accident unnatural and death by late age natural. There is no authentic definition for natural death other than our acceptance of the fact that one surely dies after a certain age even if the person has no sickness, which we call natural. In any way, death is the order of nature that every living being has to face after birth. We can only question how death is invited earlier than the time allowed by nature. While human beings toil hard to make life better and more comfortable through science, technology, and brainpower, we use all these 3 to kill. Modern states spend trillions to develop weapons and the so-called defensive system, which is practically an instrument to offend the enemies to be safe from their onslaught.

The history of the twentieth century told us how much the United States of America spent on the Manhattan Project using the brains of the world's most brilliant scientists, who worked for years. After the Soviet breakup, the world saw the secrets of their lethal preparations, which none could have imagined earlier. The Soviet secret facilities had killed thousands, without bombing. All these adventures razed thousands of people and their succeeding generations to live in misery. All these were done in the name of science.

Terrorism, which is known to have originated from dagger men called Sicarii zealots in the first century, is also an extraordinary brainwork. Ruler's inefficiency, ruthlessness or dictatorship to unaddressed famine also killed millions of their subjects. All these involve uncommon human brains. Miscalculations might not have killed so much in history. But I am afraid, the 21st century will spell doom upon our grave miscalculations.

The first pandemic of the 21st century named Covid-19 would tell the story of how our miscalculations and misjudgment rendered doom. That also showed how an invisible virus would wipe out everything human beings built over many years.

Like the nuclear disaster, industrial disasters also have taken away a large number of precious lives, directly and indirectly. Several deaths by an industrial disaster are unaccounted for even now. Despite caution and overcaution through safety rules, industrial disasters continue. There are plenty of deaths caused by pollutants that industrial complexes emit and discharge.

We need to look at it from a wider perspective not only by accidents but by exposure to the working atmosphere.

The killing sport of industrialisation is not going to stop; after all, industries determine the destiny of mankind.

The Bhopal Gas Tragedy in 1984 killed more than 16,000 people, and more than half a million people fell victim to the poisonous gas exposure. The 40 tonnes of toxic fume left a long-term impact. Many more continue to die. Beirut's ammonium nitrate tragedy in August 2020 razed almost all of the city. It was an industrial tragedy caused by a grave human error.

Before the age of technology and the discovery of the calendar system, the passage of years was counted based on the sprouting of leaves of a particular tree and the number of harvests farmers used to have. That was a wonderful natural way of counting the passage of time.

Today we live in a global village, which has become smaller and more accessible with time, thanks to the technologies that have networked all corners of the globe. It has its advantages and disadvantages. The pandemic caused by a virus is like an unchained wild animal. The infection has reached people who have maintained the most caution, practiced social distancing, and taken all the safety measures.

Today, hardly anything happens in any part of the world that people worldwide cannot find out. Thanks to the latest technologies and information media. No one can hide anything for a long time. A more unified globe means alert and aware people of all the natural and unnatural happenings.

Most people love to have relationships with others for better living comforts and happiness. These civilised and socialised human characters are not new trends. All these luxuries and necessities have now become a big burden.

Chapter 9

The Plague That Displaced Empires and Tuberculosis That Defaced Mummies

The history of bacterial and viral infections is as old as human history. It is from the very bosom of nature that every virus and bacteria originated, the same source all other living beings on the planet also emerged from. As human beings have undergone biological evolution, diseases too have accompanied them but with a solution within and around the living atmosphere. As human beings change tracks looking away from solutions within, nature also lets the virus and bacteria act on human beings.

We cannot oversee the possibility of viruses and bacteria existing in our presence. While sometimes they might be non-lethal, some infections can spin out of proportion and have a snowball effect on humankind. We have witnessed all this as a major pandemic in every century, besides a frequent, but brief, revisiting of an existing viral attack in some parts of the world. The attacks of viruses and bacteria at different times have led to the collapse of many empires, emperors, and soldiers. Historians and archaeologists have confirmed the fact after their extensive study.

In the modern age, the pandemic has led to a rearrangement of world orders. In another sense, it delivers a warning against the reckless and arrogant luxury of life - towards a compulsive change in lifestyle. The pandemic of the 21st century is going to change the world far more than what is now foreseen and predicted.

In many ways, the 21st-century pandemic is different from previous centuries' pandemics. The people of earlier centuries were not so clever, at least in terms of foraging business interests. For that reason, they were no opportunity seekers to fill the coffins. In modern days, every disaster is considered an opportunity. This is one of the major differences between the pandemic of previous centuries and the pandemic of the 21st century.

There were no systematic or formal records of the previous centuries' pandemics. The number of casualties and the extent of the epidemic impacts are only estimates. Historians and archaeologists worked hard to compile convincing evidence. Technology, in those days, was not so advanced to keep records of the epidemic victims. Another difference was the lack of awareness and preventive action. Even the modern healthcare regime in any country has been incapable of supporting epidemic control measures. New York's response to Covid-19 made the pandemic worse. Many media investigations indicated that poor management of New York leaders led to the escalation of infection and death rates. The human world was fighting a blind war not only with its human contemporaries but with an unknown and invisible enemy.

Until the end of the 18th century, the world of science didn't know about viruses. A virus was discovered more than 2 centuries after bacteria was discovered. The discovery of the tobacco mosaic virus by Ivanovski and Beijerinck in 1892 laid out the first chapter in the history of virology. Antonie van Leeuwenhoek, who fathered microbiology, wasn't a scientist but made himself a scientist through his discovery of bacteria in 1676. The microscope, which enabled humans to learn about invisible living and non-living things, was invented nearly a century before the bacterium was identified.

Some years ago, a sixth-century burial ground in Bavaria, Germany opened Pandora's box that shocked researchers. The researchers examined the skeletons of 16 corpses buried there at different times. The leftover teeth in the skeletons that did not decay were taken for DNA analysis. After a thorough study, the scientists said, without any doubt, the cause of everyone's death was the 'Justinian Plague.' The scientists, who had been exploring for many years to find the truth behind Roman emperors who ruled Western Europe, had subsequently confirmed the enemy of the emperors was none but the Plague itself. The Roman emperor Lucius Versus, along with Marcus Aurelius, also died of the Plague.

Relatively weak in front of the Roman Empire, the Burgundians, Anglers, Saxons, Jutes, and many other tribes could never have won the war with their power. However, the pandemic Plague rendered them defenceless against the Romans. Most of the Roman soldiers died of the Plague at that time giving their weak enemies an edge over the more powerful military rival. The Roman's armour was weakened due to the dismemberment of the soldiers who succumbed to the Plague. This enabled the tribes to gain dominance over their soil.

By the end of the fifteenth century, as the Plague swallowed 80 per cent of the American tribes, Eurasian settlers could build their empire in the very land that was devastated by the Plague. Thus, the 'white invaders' could build a lasting paradise for themselves in the faraway land. Later they could become indomitable to others in the world. They changed the world and stayed ahead of others in terms of socio-economic growth. It was the pandemic that had whitened the black United States of America (USA) to be the leader of the world, thanks to the dismemberment of the local tribes. This paved the way for Eurasians to settle in the land, not theirs. But the Eurasian saga did not end with their success in finding a new home on the other side of the Atlantic. The recurrence of the Plague, named the Bubonic Plague, later wiped out half of the Eurasian population in 4 years. The historians called the pandemic 'Black Death.' In the 14th century alone, it was reported that about 400 million people in Europe died of the Plague. Eurasia had to wait for another 2 centuries to see the birth of human beings equivalent to the number of 4 years of population loss. So intense was the destruction of the Plague in Eurasia.

The deadly bacteria that caused the pneumonic Plague had travelled around the world for centuries and ensured the downfall of all empires from the Roman Empire to the Mayan Empire, including Greece, Sparta, and Arabia.

The Plague won the war by ensuring the downfall of the most powerful men. It even took many years to name the bacterium Yersinia pestis (Y. Pestis), named after its discoverer Alexandre Yersin. It was only in 1895 that a study on the bacterium for developing vaccination began – long after the Plague razed empires by killing unnumbered human beings. If a pandemic could ruin emperors, there would be no need for other warfare against enemies. The world had reasonably suspected bacteria being used as bio-warfare.

In the modern age, though many dictators like the one in present China wanted to build an empire, they are not exposing their desire because they are afraid of a massive reaction from the rest of the world.

In the second wave of the Bubonic Plague, which originated in the Yunnan province of China in the second half of the nineteenth-century, India also had to pay a huge cost. An estimated 15 million people died in India in the 30-year-long Plague. China's western Yunnan province is still known as the natural reservoir of the Plague.

While Europe ruled the world until almost the middle of the last century, Plague ruled Europe more or less until the nineteenth-century. In the twentieth century, 2 world wars and other wars replaced the monstrous work of the Plague in Europe with human massacres. No one has an exact count of how many innocent and unarmed human lives perished in the wars. But the Europeans and the Americans could bury everything they suffered and build everything they wanted in a span of half a century.

For many centuries, the Plague remained a notorious killer. Molecular biologists and clinical scientists had to sweat many decades to find a breakthrough that could tackle the bacteria of the Plague before the Plague killed human beings and annihilated empires. The Plague claimed more lives than the number of lives that perished in all other devastations caused by conflicts and natural disasters put together. The world is not yet free from death by disease caused by viruses and bacteria. It has worsened now, although silently, thanks to the ruthless level of drug inducement in the name of modern treatment.

Tuberculosis (TB), a highly virulent disease, remained uncontrolled despite vaccination and targeted remedies. TB is an ongoing epidemic in history as old as human life has been on this planet. Many documents written in ancient India and China more than 3,000 years ago showed that the medical world was aware of this killer disease. Studies also reportedly showed that the Mycobacterium tuberculosis virus, which caused tuberculosis, first appeared in primitive humans millions of years ago. It stays yet with modern man, surpassing the emperors and leaders, and with aeons, it coexisted silently.

Archaeologists and forensic scientists have found that the physical degeneration of tuberculosis was evident in the forms of Egyptian mummies, 2400 years BC. Although the deformity of the skeleton exposed the story of tuberculosis, none of the Egyptian inscriptions mentioned the notorious disease prevailing in those times. TB continues to haunt human beings still. It has taken millions of lives and remains one of the top 10 causes of death, even after billions are spent on the worldwide mission of preventing it.

According to a WHO report on 24th March 2020, the worldwide death caused by TB in 2018 was 1.5 million, amounting to 15 percent of 10 million TB cases reported in that year. The number showed a high-level of mortality. The final goal of ending the TB epidemic by 2030 remains a tough dream as the alarming level of drug resistance is inevitable. TB also contributed its share to the collapse of many ancient empires, like the Plague in many names. These microbes infiltrated the cells of those who lived on this earth without discriminating against kings, courtiers, or poor slum dwellers.

Chapter 10

Nineteenth-Century Pandemic

How India was relatively safer.

As we see in history, every pandemic originated from urban centres that gradually infected rural populations. A century ago, the British colony of India had not opened up. The rural heart of India was only a secret treasure for colonial rulers. India's urban-rural divide was also huge, and inner India was wild for elite urbanites. Even while being wild and not so easily negotiable for large cities, rural India was not safe from the common epidemics seen in large cities. The Spanish flu that struck one-third of the population on this planet with a huge mortality rate a century ago had impacted India much worse than other parts of the world. The precise number of mortalities remains a mystery, and the flu left with a speculative conclusion.

The four-year-long World War I hadn't ended then. The signs of a pandemic called Spanish Influenza had begun to show up its devastating face in many parts of the world. Countries in war naturally focused more on winning the strenuous war. The pandemic was not considered an enemy by the countries where it was hit. Most of the countries' media were under censorship. In the war, Spain was neutral and Spanish media had enough freedom and bandwidth to report the alarming cases of flu. The rest of the world knew about the contagion only through Spanish media. That made the others believe the flu had Spanish origin.

The world went through a similar drill as the Spanish Flu during the COVID-19 period. More than a century after the Spanish Flu hit the world, people were again asked to stay in isolation, keep away from crowds, wash their hands very often, wear protective masks and gloves, not touch things, not spit in public and many more. The world was reeling under a severe pandemic yet again that eradicated its population largely.

The Spanish Flu Covid-19 pandemic was highly contagious with a high transmission rate. Though scientists even now could not find the origin of the flu, the infection was reported to have attacked the population of the USA and soon hit other parts of the world. The flu infected one-third of the population on the planet, killing roughly 10 per cent of the infected people. An estimated 500 million were hit and one per cent of the then-world population died in 2 years. It spread like wildfire on other continents, especially in the colonies of European powers.

Over a quarter of the Americans fell sick in those 2 years. An estimated 6.75 lakh died in the country over the period. The flu revisited the U.S. exactly a century later, striking 45 million people. About 61,000 patients succumbed to it in 1917-18. But strangely, it did not spread widely. India was safe in the early stage of the pandemic, largely because India was not as globalised as it is now. The worldwide patterns of influenza spread in 1918 adapted from reference and the Africa Centre for Strategic Studies showed at least 2 infection epicentres, the US and Europe, with relative sparing of countries such as Australia and New Zealand that could only be reached by a long sea voyage.

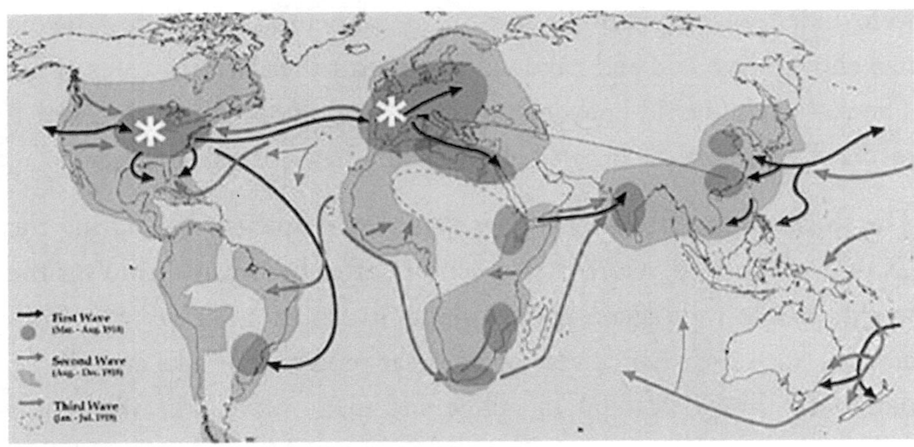

The impact of COVID as it travelled to different continents.

In June 1918, the flu landed on the Indian shore, first in Mumbai (erstwhile Bombay). The virus was suspected to have come either through cargo vessels from Europe or through the constables who were on the battlefield fighting along with the force of India's colonial masters. In India, the Spanish flu was then renamed 'Bombay Fever' as it started from Bombay, where soldiers landed after their war assignment in Europe.

It took only 2 months for it to spread all over India. Then the nation was not as openly accessible as it is now. Cities were not as dense as we see now. Social awareness about the disease was not much. Moreover, India was ruled by an outside ruler, who found the natives inferior to human beings. The pandemic thus created a terrific result. No surprise, careless handling of the infection rendered a heavy toll. The flu killed 14 million people in British-ruled India, the worst casualty in the world. God only knows if that number was right or wrong. The basis of the calculation was said to be the difference between the population census in 1911 and 1921. The population of British India fell considerably in the census of 1921 compared with the previous census. No other country was hit as badly.

The Spanish flu took a heavy death toll due to -

- Lack of effective treatment because of the unknown cause
- The cramped and unhygienic living conditions of people and animals because of the World War I scenario
- Lack of healthcare providers as most of the doctors were on the war field serving war soldiers
- The exceptional ability of the virus to duplicate itself and infect the lungs

In the past, it was not easy to know people from other corners of the world. Those who were interested in knowing about the other parts of the world were only emperors, who were willing to expand their empires, or explorers with a special interest in trade to open a new trade route. With this niche, people their cultures and lifestyle, and even diseases travelled. The ancient land of India wasn't known to have shipped any disease to the world like Egypt and China did. In the modern days, Africa, America, and China shipped infectious diseases.

However, no progress ever achieved by human beings in any sphere could stop diseases. Diseases came and went like man-made and natural disasters. Every disease was the result of unhealthy human behaviour. The broad spectrum of medical science tackled it, paving the way for another set of reactive diseases. Over a period, diseases dominated us through our different fault lines.

Chapter 11

Viruses, Which Were Found and Unfound

While we boast about our scientific achievements, we haven't stopped ourselves from worrying about infections, which led to the pandemic. Too many talks about the nature of the virus, its virulence, and predictions exposed confusion among medical experts and virologists.

Modern medicines are the inorganic solution for pain or illness. It is a shortcut that we all seek. But nature will not stop its process of creation and recreation. A virus with new strains will emerge and re-emerge in uncountable numbers. Although human beings may not be able to see most of the creations of nature. Different medical devices developed by human beings also may not support scientist's quest to see some creations.

While what is seen is tackled, millions of unseen organisms will continue to live with us harmfully or harmlessly.

How many of those who are afraid of the virus have seen the virus alive or dead? Even when it is said that the virus is lifeless outside the cellular system and an active living microbe that multiplies rapidly inside a human body, it hasn't infected everyone equally. No one has seen the virus with the naked eye. As we all will live with the legendary shape of the coronavirus, we have not seen it under a high-power microscope like a virologist or a scientist researching it.

In the first wave of COVID-19, there were certain asymptomatic cases who recovered after certain days sometimes without medicine also. But the second wave of COVID-19 brought a different strain of the virus.

The study of the character of the virus will be important in finding medical solutions to tackle it and eradicate it, making people's lives safe and fearless. However, repeating the mistake of the past, this time with more confusion, the health authorities replay the stereotypes. If the asymptomatic have no concerns, then what is the need for imposing on them the lab tests? While the majority of people were dealing with unreliable lab-test reports, imposing the lab-test on an asymptomatic patient was like soliciting the untroubled to trouble.

The health authorities should have worked out another course of action to ensure that the asymptomatic don't carry any risk. Although people were now aware of the asymptomatic category of variant too!

Patients dying of pneumonia were only confirmed a century ago when western historians, the Greek Physician, and the celebrated Father of Medicine, Hippocrates described it first in the classic era.

Sushruta Samhita, Charaka Samhita and Ashtangahridaya described many types of jwara (fever) more broadly than the description given by modern medical science.

So many interpretations about the virus have come and gone, read, and forwarded. Scientists themselves have given varying views about the virus. Some reports were unstable. Whatever the views and interpretations, the world suffered too much from it and fears created by scientists about it. We can expect many more variants to come and go and people will continue to be afraid of the virus. Over a period, they will learn to live with fear. Nature will give them the strength to live with fear and gradually adjust to it.

We are tamed to believe everything that the scientists say. We believe it religiously without daring to ask a question or even having doubts about their findings. We believe that they make no mistake, though history has proven many scientific theories were incorrect. Even in the case of diseases, use of drugs, and diagnosis also, there were plenty of revisions, after proving the earlier ones were incorrect. The best examples are the medicines recommended for the treatment of COVID-19. While some research found some medicines effective, some studies found them ineffective. Some medicines used earlier were scrapped later, finding them ineffective. But by the time a dosage was found to be ineffective, many patients died of the drugs or their side effects. The plain truths thus remained unquestioned.

Our fear of the virus made us pay until we lost our last savings. And thus, for many reasons, the COVID-19 pandemic can be considered a made-up disaster. So long we have been bullied by a virus that we have not even seen. We have been equally living in the fear created by rulers, yet, we haven't counter-questioned if the information is real or speculation. And if everything has been true? All these might appear rubbish and most might call this candid approach a ridiculous gesture. But no sensible individual has ever seen what he is always made to believe.

We must know, no animal depends on formulating medicines for their unrest or ailments. Yet, most of them still live a full life. For every discomfort, they find a solution around them. These animals have no system of research, drug development, pharmacy, or industry for medicine making. The animals don't have a research system; they exist as they do. But how we see them is they are neither civilised nor as intelligent as human beings. But will that spare them from being vulnerable to diseases? They also fall sick with equal frequency. They live a full life as allowed by nature. However, the course of human life has been distracted beyond a desirable level by modern life science. Medicines have produced more patients and too many human diseases than they are known to have saved. Medicines are good but unavoidable.

Nature has these medicines in abundance in its bosom. While taking the unnatural course, our science developed inorganic solutions. The medicines developed through the inorganic route have done more damage to human beings than was anticipated from the process of developing medicines.

We take medicines when we suffer from a fever that signifies a rise in body temperature. The medicines suppress it, though there is no need for suppressing it or controlling it with drug intervention because the body has an inbuilt system to react to pathogens - be they bacterial or viral - through self-healing. We shouldn't use any drug to control the naturally endowed mechanism of our body. We humans, need control and as we cannot control the ailment ourselves, we seek relief through a pill that is inorganically developed. And there begin our problems.

It is not the virus or bacterium that is more dangerous, but the medicine that we use for killing them before even our body prepares to expel them. The use of medicine against the virus and bacteria finally turns out to be an immunity killer, by its overreaction in our body, making the natural immune system dormant. While we ignore this fact, our fear of viruses becomes viral. And as the fear spreads, we run for cover. The human mind is easily vulnerable to fear, and it is this vulnerability that the medicine industry exploits. Ultimately, it is the virus that doesn't kill human beings, but medicine. It is not the virus that makes our lives a mess, but fear.

Our fear and modern medicines go a long way. Modern medical science and medicine have built a big world and we all live in that world, as a slave with a great degree of ignorance. And one's ignorance makes him vulnerable to being fooled.

Along with this, human being's natural weakness of following a herd mentality makes them more exploited by those who rule the world. The treatment protocols based on medicines which were claimed to show success and the protocol set for testing suspected candidates go hand-in-hand. The unproven efficacy of medicines is susceptible to health damages, but these medicines are forced on the patients. Equally terrible is the calibration of the diagnostic regime. The test hasn't been done by any wisdom of nature but by what the machine is taught by human beings with certain calibrations. These calibrations are tuned to commercial motivations.

The chemistry of the human body cannot have any standard equation, as the creation of anything by nature is not uniform. A virus, which we fear now, has inexplicable pathogenic variations. The machine, too, cannot be taught about the innumerable permutations and combinations of chemical formations happening within a human body so that it is expected to make a precise diagnosis. The test is expected to throw only a standard result in every context. That makes the test a farce for most of those who are subjected to the test. Because the machine is taught to pinpoint a suspected case based on one set of parameters that it is alerted to respond to.

All medicines used for treating corona eventually, after 3-4 months, proved to be useless and incorrect.

In the business jargon, there is this term - the prospective customer. The customer is considered a potential target for all businesses. Asymptomatic people are considered prospective customers of the medical world or what?

If a society wants to look at a person with suspicion, it can never be corrected. Tagging a patient as asymptomatic is likewise. Every diagnostic regime is also made with the same equation and thus asymptomatic cases are looked at with suspicion and are identified as being almost positive. In an asymptomatic case, the suspected infection does not make the so-called patients uncomfortable. They can stay normal even without any course of medicine. Then what is the logic behind suspecting an infection in such individuals? Of the overall reported cases of COVID-19, a vast majority of them were asymptomatic. But they are actively counted in the caseload. Similarly, the number of deaths was calculated every day, and the number was tracked by multiple agencies on a real-time basis. Before the pandemic time, no such exercise was known to have been done.

Therefore, a comparative study of the death rate between pandemic and non-pandemic times couldn't be made because there was no active death toll-count before the COVID-19 infection tracking started. But, for all sensible reasons, one with common sense can say the death rate was not lower than what was reported during the pandemic. So, is it sensible to attribute all the deaths to the novel coronavirus alone? The world of science says we hapless beings believe everything that scientists want us to believe. Only nature knows the truth.

Chapter 12

Who Thought Wuhan Wet Market Disease Would Lead to a Pandemic?

The world did not trust China. Americans and Europeans too refused to.

According to the WHO's record, it was China's Wuhan Municipal Health Commission that first reported a cluster of cases of pneumonia in its region on 31st December 2019. Four days before that, Dr Zhang Jixian from Hubei Provincial Hospital of Integrated China and Western Medicine reported to the government that the disease was caused by a novel coronavirus. Interestingly, it was on the same day, a 29-year-old doctor, Li Wenliang wrote about the virus on social media. He was a whistle-blower who was warned of spreading wrong information by the local police before he died of COVID-19 infection. In a way, the secret of the COVID-19 origin also disappeared along with the death of this whistle-blower. There were other whistle-blowers too, the media could track. However, everything was censored. The mystery behind the censorship will remain a puzzle that it originated from a country known for its mysteries.

The day after China reported the cluster of pneumonia cases to WHO, the global agency formed a three-tier Incident Management Support Team (IMST) at headquarters, regional headquarters, and country level. The aim was to deal with the pandemic outbreak. The quick action of WHO reflected its deeper understanding of the impending crisis.

Various reports suggested that the first case of Covid-19 infection was a 55-year-old unidentified person dated November 17, 2019, nearly one and a half months before China's alerting WHO. China might not have identified the deadly virus or chosen to keep the secret within the borders of the Hubei Region. China's own media report, quoting government data (South China Morning Post, Hong Kong), later said there were 266 cases of Covid-19 in 2019. Outside China and WHO, no other countries were alerted about the huge risk of the virus spreading to the entire world.

China fudged its numbers. WHO, which was unable to track through its system, could only believe what China said. The pandemic was brought under control in China with no second or third wave. The people of China removed their masks. The secret of the quick control of the pandemic, if that was true, was unknown to the world.

Though thousands were infected with the high mortality rate in Wuhan, local people in the wet market, wherefrom Covid-19 originated, were not as afraid of the pandemic as the people in New York, as well as in several European cities. China eventually locked down the wet market.

New York was devastated so badly that it shocked the entire U.S. By the end of March 2020, 50 American cities were under the rage of the pandemic. The Americans were angry with China, and so were the Europeans. U.S. Secretary of State Mike Pompeo called it the Wuhan Virus. The comment was reprimanded by Chinese officials. The counterattack of China was of the worst style as it sought unreasonable details from the U.S., where the first case of Covid-19 was spotted 3 weeks after China sent its alert to WHO. An American's Wuhan visit made him sick 4 days after his return. Thus, Washington got its first case. The second case was reported from Chicago, that too from a Wuhan returnee. Every Wuhan visitor carried back the virus that eventually devastated the world.

By April 2020, the entire U.S. began to toss over the pandemic, with the cases peaking at over 11,000 a day. By the end of September, close to 33,000 people died of the pandemic and a record half a million caseload. Since June 2020, the number of cases reported fell heavily. The city was shaken for 100 days before people began to go for jobs in early June. By the end of 2020, the U.S. report of infection was in alarming numbers. The country was helpless as the new U.S. government inherited the worst Covid-19 legacy. The second wave was even more terrific.

China tried hard to misguide the world with its lies. It tried every possible way to wash its dirty hands secretly and made false confessions for release. But the world was not ready to believe what China wanted to say. China's official foreign ministry spokesperson, Zhao Lijian, tried to lay blame on the U.S. by discovering an argument that the virus was brought by the U.S. army. China tried to scuttle the world's call for an investigation into the origin of the virus with its immature counterattacks.

Many cities in Italy were shattered badly, thanks to the high volume of traffic between China and Italy. The Milan Exhibition Centre in Italy, running well over a quarter of a million square feet, was converted into an intensive care facility with thousands of beds and ventilators. Almost every major European city was ravaged by the pandemic in the biting cold winter.

The world had acquired new hopes at the turn of the millennium. The disease management capability of the generally haughty developed economies in the world, which used to indulge in dictating standards for developing countries like India, was put to the test. Nearly 2 years after the pandemic, everything around the world changed.

Chapter 13

The Unplugged Viral Fault Lines

Rumours, unreasonable interpretations, unverified news, and contradictory statements were the commonly seen information in the days of the pandemic. The pandemic was not a very serious virus-induced pandemic but made to be more excessively serious by news which went viral through the media to add to many other mismanagements.

I mentioned in the early part of this book, every day hundreds of news stories about Covid-19 appeared and spread virally like wildfire. Some were new findings; sometimes baseless and sometimes contradictory. Covid-19 news dominated the pages of newspapers around the world in the entire year of 2020 and most of 2021. Publications carried repeated cover stories on Covid-19 with new dimensions. Media analysis of Covid-19 information from economic, political, and scientific perspectives. The media, while entirely loss-making during the lockdown period, came up grabbing people's attention and celebrating in the form of story after story. In the early days, the reports were based on endless miseries of people in countries where the virus was said to have a field day. The pictures of chaos in hospitals, streets, workplaces, etc. became sensational. At the fag-end of the year 2020, the focus was shifted to the vaccine launch, preparations for inoculation, production tasks, shipment challenges, etc. The reports of discussions between vaccine makers and the government, emergency approval, cold chain infrastructure for transportation, pricing, priority groups, etc. filled the media spaces. As the inoculation started, the public fear and adverse impacts found space in the media.

As said before, we are living in a global village, which is becoming smaller with every passing day due to technology and connectivity worldwide. And so is the reason Covid-19 became infamous, though the infection later proved to be not more than flu. After all, making the world a village has its advantages and disadvantages.

The worst impact of the sudden lockdown announcement came on the migrant workers in India. They were left without protection against the virus. Most faced hunger or homelessness if they could not work.

The heart-wrenching scene of migrant workers leaving cities to return to their hometowns was one of the most difficult times India has seen. Without any means of transportation, these workers undertook a long and dangerous journey on foot, often without food or water. Many of them didn't make it to their destination.

Although the government advertised the 'Vande Bharat Mission' to fly back Indians stranded abroad, the locals suffered. Hundreds of people camped out at railway stations hoping for a train.

At a quarantine centre in Uttar Pradesh's Gorakhpur district, 17-year-old Baliram Kumar, who had walked from Bangalore over 25 days, says, "I've got cuts and bruises all over my feet," he said wearily into the phone, a day after he'd finally arrived back home in his village. "I had shoes, but they were no good after a while. I'm so tired. My whole body is aching." The journey had turned them into nocturnal creatures, and by the end, many were barely able to walk. "We walked from 3 am to 10 am and rested during the day," he said.

Vinod Yadav, a 20-year-old man, was quarantined in Katihar district, Bihar. He travelled for 27 days from Bangalore before finally arriving in his village. Part of his journey was made on foot, and during the sweltering late-May heat, he and his companions took rests for 4-5 hours during the day. Otherwise, they would walk all day and night.

As the COVID-19 pandemic affected people worldwide, there has been an influx of myths and untruths surrounding the topic. The pandemic created more headlines than just the right news. There were simultaneous misinformation and rumours.

Below, we debunk some of the most common myths currently circulating on social media and beyond:

Myths

- WHO busts some myths that were making rumours during the COVID-19 pandemic.
- Spraying and introducing bleach or another disinfectant into your body WILL NOT protect you against COVID-19 and can be dangerous.
- Exposing yourself to the sun or temperatures higher than 25°C DOES NOT protect you from COVID-19.
- Drinking alcohol does not protect you against COVID-19 and can be dangerous.
- Water or swimming does not transmit the COVID-19 virus.
- Vitamin and mineral supplements cannot cure COVID-19.
- Touching a communal bottle of alcohol-based sanitiser will not infect you.
- It is safer to frequently clean your hands and not wear gloves.
- The amount of alcohol-based sanitiser you use matters.

WHO has on its site a dedicated page where it was asking for people to report misinformation about Covid as a part of the 'Stop the Spread Campaign' started in May-June 2020.

The article by BBC titled 'Coronavirus: The human cost of virus misinformation' says, "A BBC team tracking coronavirus misinformation has found links to assaults, arsons, and deaths." And experts say the potential for indirect harm caused by rumours, conspiracy theories, and bad health information could be much bigger.

The Case of Hydroxychloroquine

According to a BBC article, Hydroxychloroquine may have the potential to fight the virus - but as research continues, it remains unproven. The World Health Organisation halted its use in trials after a recent study suggested it could increase the risk of patients dying from Covid-19.

Speculation about its effectiveness started circulating online in China in late January. Media organisations, including Chinese state outlets, tweeted out old studies where it was tested as an anti-viral medicine.

In Nigeria, hospital admissions from hydroxychloroquine poisoning provoked Lagos state health officials to warn people against using the drug.

During the pandemic, this proved more negative than positive as foul goes viral faster than facts, faster than even the viral infection could spread. That was the reason isolated cases of vaccine reaction became viral and such reports made people reluctant to go for the jab. These rumours were certainly contributing to the fear and chaos while the shattering second wave further terrified people. Eventually, the prediction of a third wave made people indifferent to fear, but vaccines were mandatory, and the government accelerated the rush for the vaccine in India.

Chapter 14

Misfired Lockdown

News Headlines in India during May 2021, the peak of the lockdown:

- *Bengal restricts the number of invitees to weddings to 50 as COVID cases rise. It has also given directives to shut down malls, gyms, beauty parlours, and restricts gatherings amid rising Covid cases.*
- *COVID-19: Haryana orders closure of all shops by 6 pm, bans non-essential gatherings.*
- *Covid-19: New restrictions in Maharashtra ban gatherings; schools, colleges to remain shut.*
- *As Covid-19 cases increase, Karnataka restricts large gatherings.*
- *Omicron scare: Delhi Govt bans social gatherings and celebrations ahead of Christmas & New Year.*

The socio-economic impact of the lockdown was severe. The economic package and free ration supply had limitations, though the measures might have brought some relief.

The government could have planned the lockdown with better prudence. As the lockdown began to be eased when the Covid-19 numbers were at their peak. As the economy began to rebound, people began to see a course of relief. That proved that even without the lockdown, the pandemic could have been controlled.

No other country in the world had seen such a strict nationwide lockdown as India had been put under. We were the worst hit developing economy.

I still believe India has taken so many actions in a hurry, too early without sufficient thought and planning. In a democracy, an elected government is accountable to people for actions and failures equally. Therefore, it is insensible for anyone to expect the government to keep watching for a longer time to take any action with better prudence.

However, we need to make an impact assessment of the blind orders to lock down the entire country, free ration distribution to 800 million people, cash transfers to poor women, 20 trillion worth of economic refuelling, liberal loans, and the longer moratorium on repayment, etc., with a thorough realistic sense. So many policy plans have been put on hold. Infrastructure development, disinvestment plans, bad loan recovery plans of banks, and so many other actions were left halfway.

A pandemic could do anything worse than war could. We could read what was reported as the 2020-21 first-quarter GDP. Though free ration was not supposed to fuel economic growth, the cash transfers to create demands, liberal loans to restart small businesses, and moratoriums as relief measures were supposed to fire the economy in the long run. The construction segment was contracted by more than 50 per cent. The segment was completely dormant, except for those segments where force majeure was not applicable. Even in those segments where force majeure was not applicable, the plights of workers led to shutting the worksite. Things did not change even by early September.

The lockdown was an advantage for lazy people whose incomes somehow had been steady. Lawmakers never suffered from any disaster.

But they were driven by the interests of the highly influential class. The highly influential class inherently can convert every disadvantage into an advantage. They could turn the tide of the pandemic to their advantage.

Over time, people were tired of sitting at home isolated and were now coming out on the streets. The Pandemic became endemic. Masks were gradually disappearing from people's faces. In proportion to the traffic density on roads, business sentiments didn't pick up. Hotels and restaurants were still largely closed. Construction sites remained shut even in the second wave. There were talks of strict lockdown again in the second wave, but no state was ready for such an adventure. People were not even ready to sit at home for fear of their job loss.

The pandemic has led to several months of changes to our routines which may have resulted in changes to our behaviour that will persist long after the pandemic is over. According to Wiebke Bleidorn, a personality change lab researcher at the University of California, Davis, "This may lead to new norms, which may over time also shape our personalities."

The lockdown may have turbo-charged a phenomenon known as 'The Michelangelo Effect,' which refers to how we're more likely to develop into the kind of person we want to be if we're with a close romantic partner who supports our aspirations and encourages us to behave accordingly.

For people with a supportive partner, the lockdown period might have been a chance for personal growth. But for those stuck indoors in an unhappy relationship or being harassed by their children, the effects on their personality are sure to have been negative. And what about those people who were left completely isolated on their own during the lockdown?

If this forced solitary confinement provoked intense loneliness, we might predict, based on earlier research into loneliness and personality, an adverse effect on people's traits, in terms of increased neuroticism and an enforced reduction in extroversion. However, the lockdown data available to date paints a picture of human resilience.

From the last century's history, we could learn the fact that India was the worst victim of pandemics. India, be it under British rule or its own elected governments, had paid a bigger price every time. We need to ponder over it seriously. Before the onset of the monsoon of 2020, some experts predicted the number of Covid-19 cases to soar to an alarming size. In the early days, it was unimaginable to foresee daily new cases as high as 97,000. But that was a reality.

Ultimately, the shocking numbers didn't shock anyone by the time the number hit the roof. People learned to live with a high number of cases without any shock or fear. Mid-way through the monsoon, the number of cases reported in India reached closer to 2 million. In September 2020, every 15 days added one million cases, with equally fast recoveries, thereby the active caseload remained stagnant at around a million and below.

Modern medicine couldn't find any solution to chain the virus, despite its intense efforts, tight guidance as per its directive, stopping all activities and constant changing medical protocols.

We humans never stopped boasting about the great achievements of modern methods of treatment. We have always used technology to complement our work on opening new methods of treatment. Yet, we have reached nowhere. We have lost a war to the virus, which is too invisible a lifeless particle said to conquer our cellular system. In my first book, published barely 6 months before the outbreak of the pandemic, I dwelt on how mischievously we play with nature. Certainly, one day we will pay for this mischief.

Yet, we are regulated with insensibility to make us follow a protocol set by national and world authorities virtually enslaving us for our ignorance and freedom. Here we are paying heavily for infringing truths. Maybe, for this reason, the countries which boast of freedom, human development, healthcare, etc., paid more heavily. But we haven't learned anything. Instead, we preferred to grapple with a herd mentality.

On April 1st, 2020, the Narendra Modi led Union government announced a nationwide lockdown in India due to the outbreak of Covid-19. The country had 618 cases at the time. A year later to the date, India was preparing for the Kumbh Mela - one of the world's largest religious congregations - despite having 3 million active Covid cases and a total tally of over 11 million.

Despite experts across the country cautioning against holding the event, the administration turned a deaf ear to those appeals. Even at the event itself, state government advertisements paid lip service to Covid protocols, but it was clear to all but the most credulous that it wouldn't be possible to observe the protocol at this mela of millions.

Tirath Singh Rawat, Chief Minister of Uttarakhand, declared: "Faith will overcome the fear of Covid-19." Pity, it couldn't stave off the disease too.

The Kumbh Mela is a holy event for Hindus that takes place over the course of a month. This time it was taking place amid a surge in COVID-19 cases, with the daily case count crossing the 200,000 mark. Nevertheless, neither the Union health ministry nor the state government had taken steps to stop the Kumbh. It took Prime Minister Modi 17 days to request people to participate symbolically for the rest of the event. The Union home ministry could have stopped the event by invoking the Disaster Management Act (DMA), but it was instead chosen to look the other way. On April 27, nearly 25,000 people participated in the holy dip, with barely a mask in sight.

As the pandemic expanded, we put off the light and chose to grope in the dark and tried to reach an easy method of lockdown. So many medicines, which were not targeted for Covid-19, were tested on patients. Many patients died because of the ineffectiveness of the medicine given to them. Some Covid-19 patients died not because of Covid-19 but of other diseases, including heart failure.

We couldn't control the epidemic because our fear and hypochondria were nature's engineering work. Humans fall into their self-dug trap. Like Bhasmasura who trapped Lord Shiva with the boon he received from Shiva.

Finally, India became the world's worst hit by being one of the 3 countries to have the highest number of cases.

The only hope was that India was called to be the world's biggest pharmacy, as British Prime Minister Boris Johnson said. When Covid-19 broke out, India had great optimism of being resistant to the infection. Initially, we even boasted about the slow spread of infection compared with the cases reported in many European countries and the U.S. Nonetheless, by the mid of March 2020, we took a sudden turn after astonishingly watching what was reported from other countries. Then India ran for cover in panic seeing the worrisome number.

Chapter 15

An Ordeal Called Modern Medical Science

While modern medicines couldn't save a vulnerable class of patients, traditional medicines saved immeasurable millions. While roads were blocked and offices were closed, farmers braved the pandemic to feed people. Indian villages didn't fear the virus but feared the impact of the pandemic.

We have seen the explosion of the pandemic, deaths by it, fear of people, and failure of the medical fraternity in managing the amplified flu. One can assertively say that Covid-19 seems to have tested the capability of modern medical science.

There hasn't been any direct remedy for controlling the rapidly infecting virus, yet some medicines were administered for treating the infection. And this has been a questionable decision. While most patients recovered through these medicines, there is a percentage of people who also succumbed to them. A larger number of patients with no symptoms didn't even need medicine for recovery and many who have taken these medications wait to face the after effects of it.

Remedies the modern medical fraternity may not accept, but India's traditional home remedy against viral infection has been very effective. Many practitioners of modern medicine have secretly admitted this, some even openly. At the same time, it was seen that no drugs could eliminate the killer virus and save infected people. Our immune response system could tranquillise the virus entering the body either with the support of supplementary medicines, by herbal treatment, or naturally. Therefore, vaccination becomes necessary only when all drugs fail, and when clinical attempts to deliver a drug to fail.

Let's remember the pandemic scenario. The atmosphere was inexplicably horrendous when the number of infections was in the hundreds. Contrarily, as the numbers grew, people grew immune to the fear. Schools were closed unprecedentedly for many months since the lockdown began. Children did not go to school for almost a full academic year 2020-21, and the first half of the year 2021-22 wasn't different either. Airports and seaports too were shut. Had these traveller's emerging points closed when Covid-19 was reported from China, the pandemic could have been curtailed from its widespread. As the lockdown was announced, all roads were blocked, and state borders were closed everywhere in India. Shops and factories pulled down their shutters indefinitely, and all of a sudden. Labourers walked thousands of kilometres to return to their hometowns to their shelter while facing the uncertainty of the future.

The book mentions the horrendous scenario of the lockdown in subsequent chapters of this book. Places of worship closed the gates of gods against devotees prayer. Gods were safe from the people, who were spreading the infection.

The unseen virus made the world run in fear and panic. And that was not all. The United Nations agencies had warned that more than 35 million people in the Asia-Pacific region are going to be hungry as the pandemic washed away jobs. Combined with this, the rise in food prices would add to their woes.

In India, food prices did not go up much, as being an agricultural country, our hardworking farmers defied the regime of lockdown and worked relentlessly. The irony was they couldn't afford to sit at home. In many places, local administrations were ruthless, and despite that, the farmers continued their farming. The farming community was not infected, as most of the Indian villages remained aloof from the pandemic fear. Therefore, India did not go hungry, as our farmers braved the pandemic to feed the people.

The strict lockdown forced people to be safe from the pandemic, while Covid-19 remained without targeted medicine all through the months. It saw more than 120 drug companies sprinting on a fast track for vaccine development. In haste, some medicines were re-profiled without any proof of their efficacy and disposed of their stocks, probably an unsuccessful trial on patients.

The first major defensive mechanism was social distancing and quarantining the victims and suspicious victims. The other popular solution was home remedies and precautions. The second solution gained popularity and eventually saved a large number of patients, thanks to the remedy of nature.

We saw the risk of modern medical science failing miserably in tackling the virus because most of those who have undergone the treatment through exposure to untargeted medicines became victims of other serious disorders. The logic of developing modern medicine with wisdom has failed as the use of certain drugs led to serious complications. As a standard protocol of Allopathy, the modern healthcare sector is not supposed to develop any medicine which carries a risk of any kind. That is the very reason a drug development takes a long period of trial, as each drug is supposed to prove 100 percent safe in patients. Whereas most of the death from Covid-19 happened because of drug complications.

The entire world has helplessly stood as a mute spectator throughout the pandemic's vaccine developing and testing stage. It was obvious that there is some kind of business motive than a logical approach. Business intelligence took precedence over the ethics of the medical industry.

With states going lax on contact tracing and tracking of positive cases, the virus was left to spread unchecked. In 2020, Indian authorities widely used the T3 protocol (test, treat, track) in the battle against Covid-19. However, in 2021, none of the states most affected by the second wave appears to be following it, with mandatory quarantining also falling by the wayside. This is a major factor behind the rapid spread of cases in the second wave.

"The T3 protocol was very effective in the months of April to August," said an official from the health department. "With the recent surge in cases, we need every hand on deck right now, and unfortunately do not have the manpower to conduct contact tracing. Although the home ministry published guidelines on March 23 asking states to strictly follow the T3 protocol, some state officials have decided to suspend tracing programmes. We are testing aggressively, doing around 60,000 tests per day," they said.

Despite being one of the states hardest hit by the second wave of Covid-19, Maharashtra's contact tracing efforts have been dismal. According to state health department officials, there is no system in place to ensure contact tracing of the almost 4 million people in home quarantine as of May 2.

In an attempt to improve the situation, the state launched the 'Chase the Virus' programme in June 2020, which aimed at tracing at least

20 people who had come in contact with each Covid-positive person. However, it is unclear how successful this programme has been so far.

Even states that did well in the first wave of the pandemic were faltering. In Bihar, the speed at which new cases had spread overwhelmed the medical infrastructure. By May 2, the state had over 100,000 active cases, shifting the priority from tracing to treatment. The state was struggling to keep up with the demand for hospital beds and oxygen cylinders.

Ideally, as everyone desires, medical scientists should have a clear picture of the nature of the virus and knowledge of its pathogenic character. Every virology lab in the world tried to study Covid-19, but with vastly varying results. Some of them even came up with confusing conclusions.

The vast majority of the victims could save themselves through home remedies and traditional medicines wherever there have been parallel cases of common cold and cough due to climate changes unless tested positive for Covid-19, where antibiotics and ibuprofen have been supported.

In the initial days of the lockdown, all dispensaries and most hospitals that were not designated for the treatment of Covid-19 were closed. Pharmacies, which used to sell painkillers and some categories of antibiotics, were asked not to sell these items. That decision was a denial of people's right to seek treatment from dispensaries and hospitals in their neighbourhood. Then people with common colds and coughs were compelled to undergo Covid-19 tests. There were many cases of Covid-19 positive test reports proven to be fake in the subsequent tests or tests from parallel labs. Such instances shocked people and led to their distrust of the medical system. Many people became prisoners of the Covid-19 protocol. Many people died of wrong treatments, which baffled the public and resulted in a loss of their confidence in practitioners of modern medicine. Wrong pandemic management, combined with non-targeted medicine used on a trial basis, intensified the Covid-19 crisis, ultimately adding to public fear.

Anyone who kept a close watch on the pandemic management and its tight protocols would understand that it was the straightjacket approach that had killed more people, infected a much larger number of people, devastated a lion's share of surviving urbanites with job loss, and ultimately destabilised the national and global economy. The failure was all-pervading. When people violated the lockdown, they could contribute to the economy.

Farmers are the best example. It may take years for the entire world and much longer for Europe and the U.S. to return to the pre-Covid-19 level peak growth. I see the so-called pandemic only as a tester of modern medical science and the commonsense of those who rule the world. In the ordeal, both of them failed but left behind a big stain on human history. Though it may sound paradoxical, the progress of science witnessed an erosion of human wisdom. That was evident from the decision to implement a rigid treatment system, while other better avenues were there.

Many states have cited a lack of manpower as a critical problem, but technology could help even with less workforce. The Union government's Arogya Setu mobile app was widely promoted during the first wave of Covid-19. Those who had been tested for Covid-19 were expected to upload the results onto the app, reducing the need for manual data entry by workers. However, there is very little compliance, if any, with these requirements now, which defeats the purpose of having the technology in the first place.

Chapter 16

That Created a Global Crisis!

Someone seemingly wanted people to live in fear and be cautious always. Initially, confident India eventually counted Covid-19 cases in millions. The second wave was the worst, but fortunately, sooner people moved out of their mental trap of fear. The pandemic spoke of the interesting story of the developed world's shocking vulnerability and poor countries' brave resistance.

The world kept watching when China, Europe, and America began to sneeze. The winter of 2020 was colder for Europe and America, wherefrom the world had to listen to some chilling reports. Their boastful healthcare systems had collapsed as the pandemic held roots.

India at the early stage saw its massive population being safe and calculated a remote chance of making it a pandemic in the densely populated sub-continent. The world knew if developed nations like Europe and America suffered so badly, then there was no footing for underdeveloped or developing nations. However, the Covid-19 spark in India could make vested interests achieve their goal. Our lawmakers should have been a bit cautious of it and stood prepared for managing it more efficiently, instead of stumbling on others tunes. When the summer of 2020 set in India, the fear began to spread as the virus was given a larger-than-life image. The fear was amplified to bring everything to a halt.

We humans sometimes follow a herd mentality. Our lawmakers were terribly perplexed before Covid-19 cases appeared in double digits. At the end of April 2020, more than a month after the complete lockdown, India reported only 1823 Covid-19 cases.

The lockdown was enforced so strictly that none dared to step out. That number was not something to worry about. But an atmosphere was built to frighten the public like a calamity was going to strike. The only calamity that struck was the uncalculated aftermath of the illogical lockdown. Millions of self-employed people were locked inside their homes to see each penny they earned depleted and had no hope of recovering their losses or even earnings. No one had an exact picture of what would happen but depended on the authorities guess and projections. And all the projections went wrong.

The infected number multiplied towards the end of summer. When India's Covid-19 cases touched 5000, a prediction of crossing the number into lakhs and millions was only an improbability. However, the numbers escalated having given the character of the infection and testing method. People were subjected to RT-PCR tests which was a trauma in itself for some.

What is the RT-PCR?

The nose swab PCR test for COVID-19 is a highly accurate and reliable test for diagnosing the virus. A positive test result means you are infected with COVID-19, while a negative result indicates that you probably did not have the virus at the time of the test or at all.

PCR, or polymerase chain reaction, is a test used to detect the presence of genetic material from a specific organism - such as a virus. Even after you are no longer infected, PCR can sometimes still detect fragments of the virus.

According to the CDC, it's possible to have coronavirus and experience little to no symptoms. Additionally, those who do experience symptoms may not have all of the symptoms listed above.

A healthcare provider will use a swab to collect a sample of respiratory material from your nose for the COVID-19 PCR test. Swabs are soft-tipped and long with a flexible stick that is inserted into your nose. There are different types of nose swabs, including nasal swabs that collect a sample immediately inside your nostrils and nasopharyngeal swabs that go further into the nasal cavity for collection.

PCR tests are very sensitive and can detect even small amounts of the SARS-CoV-2 virus. This means that you may continue to test positive for the virus even after you have recovered from COVID-19 and are no longer contagious. So, if you have had COVID-19 in the past, you may still test positive, even though you can't spread the virus to others.

Government Mandates

According to government and airport authorities mandates, only passengers who are fully vaccinated against Covid-19, have recovered from the virus, or can show a negative RT-PCR report from the last 72 hours were allowed to travel and enter certain states. In case a passenger doesn't have any of these, RAT (Rapid Antigen Test) for Covid-19 was mandated before entry.

The Bombay High Court upheld a circular issued by the Mumbai Port Trust (MPT) which required unvaccinated employees to undergo

RT-PCR tests every 10 days. The court said that the testing mandate is a reasonable restriction on their fundamental rights.

What causes false positive results?

The RT-PCR test is very accurate. If someone does not have the infection, there is a high chance the test will be negative. On the other hand, if someone is infected with the virus, there is a high chance the test will be positive.

Although the test is quite specific, there is still a slim chance that someone who isn't infected could test positive, referred to as a 'false positive.'

The most common reasons for a false positive result are laboratory error or cross-reaction with something other than SARS-CoV-2. Examples of laboratory errors include incorrect sample testing, clerical error, cross-contamination from another individual's positive sample, or issues with the reagents used in the test like chemicals, enzymes, or dyes. A person who has previously had COVID-19 and recovered might also test positive on a subsequent test.

The false-negative rate for SARS-CoV-2 RT-PCR testing can vary significantly: with the highest rate occurring within the first 5 days after exposure (up to 67%) and the lowest rate on day 8 after exposure (21%).

Even though several people have tested negative for Covid-19, they may still be showing symptoms, or their family members have tested positive. These doubts are obvious for people staying in close-knit families. They have tested negative for the virus in rapid or RT-PCR tests despite being close to infected people.

As scepticism around rapid antigen tests continues to grow, state government data shows that 0.17% of samples tested in Maharashtra have failed to identify the Sars-Cov-2 virus. This means that 3.4% of all tests in Mumbai suburbs have come back as false negatives - the highest rate in the state.

Since the end of June, 675,035 individuals have undergone antigen testing. Of those who tested negative for the virus, 4,235 symptomatic individuals had to undergo a confirmatory reverse transcription polymerase chain reaction (RT-PCR) test - considered the gold standard.

These high false-negative rates are cause for concern, especially as more and more people are relying on rapid antigen tests to give them quick results. It's important to remember that these tests are not 100% accurate.

Even though it was a relief for government officials, health experts claim that the 'abnormally low' false-negative numbers don't show the real infection rate. This means that people who were caught in this dilemma were subject to unwanted quarantine and plight at the hands of officials for data that was not in people's control.

In this ordeal, even the scientists were confused. In many cases, test results were erratic, leaving room for doubt. A negative case was also counted as Covid-positive, by mistake, non-standardisation, or confusion.

It was difficult to minutely differentiate the common cold and Covid-19 in most cases. In some cases, it was positive in the first test report and soon the same case turned out to be negative in the second test report. This rapid shift in the test reports questioned the efficiency, authenticity, and reliability of the test or the method used for it.

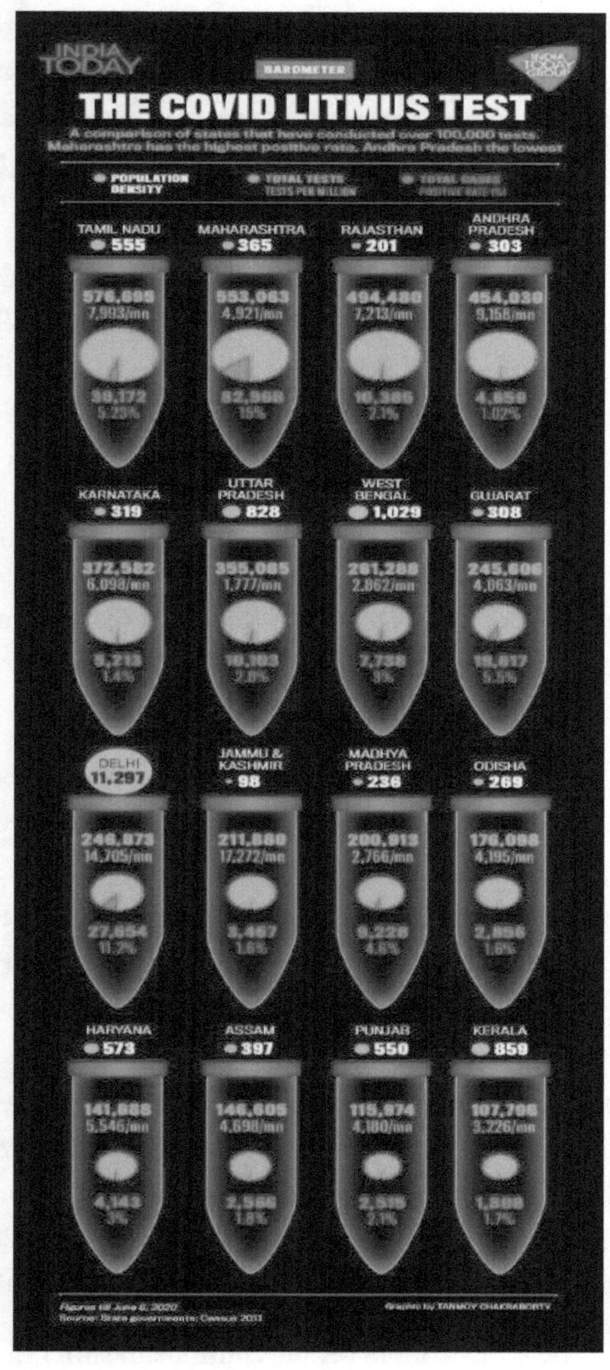
INDIA TODAY
BAROMETER
THE COVID LITMUS TEST
A comparison of states that have conducted over 100,000 tests. Maharashtra has the highest positive rate. Andhra Pradesh the lowest
POPULATION DENSITY
TOTAL TESTS
TESTS PER MILLION
TAMIL NADU 555
7,993/mn
MAHARASHTRA 365
553,063
4,921/mn
RAJASTHAN 201
494,480
7,213/mn
ANDHRA PRADESH 303
9,158/mn
KARNATAKA 319
6,098/mn
UTTAR PRADESH 828
1,777/mn
WEST BENGAL 1,029
2,862/mn
GUJARAT 308
4,063/mn
DELHI 11,297
14,705/mn
JAMMU & KASHMIR 98
17,272/mn
MADHYA PRADESH 236
2,766/mn
ODISHA 269
4,195/mn
HARYANA 573
141,888
5,546/mn
ASSAM 397
4,698/mn
PUNJAB 550
4,180/mn
KERALA 859
3,226/mn

How does it happen? Is the test kit not fit enough to read the presence of the virus in the second case, or has the first test report in such cases failed to make a correct reading? Or, we may have to say the virus becomes inactive in some people in 3 days, in the interim of the first and second test.

Somehow, the case predictions proved to be correct. But India then required an emergency focus on the economy, which was failing more seriously than treating the Covid-19 victims. We counted the numbers more seriously without paying attention to what the count meant. The count could only be held onto the fear of the masses, and normal life was locked.

On 16th June 2020, when the overall number of cases in India was below 11,000, Times Fact-India Outbreak Report projected India's active cases to reach 2.6 lakhs on 15th July 2020. People were aghast at such a projection and found it unbelievable.

Much had been discussed about the novel Coronavirus over several months. Many studies were carried out on the character of the virus worldwide and deployed cutting-edge technology to split and analyse the pathogen. Billions have been kept aside for pouring into the study, ultimately to develop vaccines and medicines for treatment that would make the drug industry significantly rich. Many large companies intensified their search for a solution and in a hurry introduced ineffective medicines to treat mild, moderate, and severe cases, without studying the long-term impact of their uses. Several hundred thousand people died, and millions were recuperating across the world. Though the death toll began to fall in the second half of October 2020, the world seemingly stood worried about the economic and medical aftershocks.

No one knows how many more people continue to suffer ill health after their recoveries. All through the pandemic, everything went beyond all predictions. While the erratic nature of Corona perplexed scientists, the economic situation confused economists, who were yet to come to terms with serious issues faced by people at the bottom of the pyramid.

But was India confident of controlling the infection numbers? Or was the country riding on fear? Did fear have any basis? Over-confident India never anticipated the Covid-19 victim's number to be above 10,000 initially. But the number rose sixteen-fold in a matter of weeks, far beyond projected. By the end of June 2021, close to 31 million people were infected in India and the situation remained grim even at the end of the 15th month of the lockdown.

The only hope was accelerated recovery with a choice of home remedies, no government intervention, or compulsion of any local health authority. Everything appeared like a ploy, and yet people chose to brave it. As people were gradually getting used to Covid-19 and adjusting to the pandemic, the government controls made normal life more difficult.

Why is the mortality rate even among co-morbid cases different? Why is it less in India compared with the cases in western countries where the mortality rate is said to be very high? Is it because of India's efficient medical system or lifestyle adhering to traditional foods? There is also a significant inconsistency in transmission within the family of a victim. In most cases, all the family members of the first victim were not infected. There was a vast difference in the infection level. Doctors may call it a variation in immunity level, but what about the toddlers related to the victims? In many cases, toddlers tested positive while the mother tested negative. It means a person with strong immunity is highly resilient to the infection, yet the infection is considered dreadful. People's behaviour during the pandemic had changed such that all members of the infected person's family were looked at with the stigma of being from the patient's family and thus untouchable. These and many more doubts are subjects of a broad-level debate.

There may be certain things some scientists must have known but are unwilling to share as scientists work on the unsaid truths. The world has seen many diseases, both bacterial and viral, with no medicines in recent years. Rather, none of the recently identified diseases has targeted medicines. Even the SARS category has no medicines so far. The medicines which were developed for some of these diseases had failed. Out of these, some drugs have found their way into Covid-19 patients without establishing their efficacies.

Despite this, the transmission could be contained, and the disease was managed to some extent. In the case of Covid-19 also, despite having no medicine, patients were treated successfully.

The mortality rate was not as high as Ebola or Nipa, or for that matter, the widely common dengue fever or malaria. All these diseases, including the contagious ones, are treated by almost every class of hospitals. That way, every hospital could treat Covid-19 too if permitted. At the same time, we classified the hospitals for the treatment of Covid-19, curtailing the overall capacity of hospitalisation and comfort of patients, especially in densely populated cities. What a preparation failure.

In Mumbai, there were reports of patients being treated under flyovers after the full-capacity utilisation of a big Covid hospital. Private hospitals have enough facilities, which were remaining idle even when they were ready to manage the crisis. But the system demanded specialised Covid hospitals, and people had to oblige as derogatory as being treated under a flyover with no proper sanitation and hygiene as well as in the sweltering heat of the summers.

A hospital is meant for taking in every patient seeking treatment. For the sake of argument, one can say the transmission rate of Covid-19 is higher. Yet, there would be no hospital which could be careless of containing the threat of infections they faced. If a hospital can treat a disease, for sure, it is also able to manage the contagion. The world has seen diseases haunting humanity for centuries, which were later defeated with the development of vaccines, medicines, and self-control. There were diseases that had changed the equation of empires and dominions. There are diseases that have medicines and vaccines and are yet known to kill human beings. Several hundred thousand people die of tuberculosis (TB) every year, despite having effective medicines and vaccination. Therefore, Covid-19 even after the discovery of medicines and vaccination may not disappear. We have to live with it. A medical scientist may call this phenomenon herd immunity. But the devastation left behind remains a serious mental and economic devastation.

The policemen were helpless but compelled to remain in their uniform in every inhospitable situation. That led to the systematic deterioration of their health. I met many policemen working in Navi Mumbai under hostile conditions in May, June, and July 2020. They were working in a danger zone; so, I thought, it was our duty to support them. They needed proper counselling, handholding, supply of medicines, and protection of healthcare, which could have helped them resist infections, stay mentally strong, and reduce their stress.

However, they didn't get any of these. The media had forgotten all these since these uniformed men were not commercially beneficial for them or their interests. These were the social issues that our Fourth Estate considered a foreign space. The government was busy correcting comments, balancing counter-comments, and looking for many ways to survive, as the crisis deprived people of their normal livelihood. Everyone was searching for someone to pass the buck and pull on as long as the foul show ended. Where will we reach was a question we had all left to the almighty to answer.

Chapter 17

Distortion of Facts and Instability in Findings

Developments of vaccines could be marked as important milestones in human history. The attempt showed the scientific prowess of human beings. Many of the attempts had a social aim too. For that very reason, vaccine development wasn't a business at one point in time. For that reason, by the 1980s, vaccine makers became financially sick. Today, overzealous vaccine makers rush to the finishing point with huge calculations. First, it was a single-dose vaccine and then it was increased to 2 doses, and then the booster. Only time can tell us how many more doses there will be!

Much has happened in modern medicine and medical research as an industry in the last quarter of a century. Innovation in the healthcare system, sophisticated diagnostic technologies, setting parameters for pathological factors and biochemistry, etc., could lead to early diagnosis of diseases and making curative plans. However, everything that has business significance has ultimately been ruthless, of course with its necessary results. An innovative way of treatment, technologies for managing complicated medical procedures, and the development of new drugs for new indications have induced great confidence in patients.

All these are welcome as long as these achievements ensure better quality and a longer lifespan. Nonetheless, there are observers who have made an analysis of how the crazy industrialisation of the healthcare system created more patients, and in its wake impacted the quality of life. Often, seeing what happens around us and how unsatisfied people are, modern medicines cannot be openly boasted as a great achievement. Every medicine has minor or major side effects. While some medicines for chronic indications do not treat sickness but enable the patient to live with the disease as long as the person's other organs can sustain it. Even then, people blindly believe modern medicines had magical power in treating them.

A magical belief has made medicines our lifelong friends. The so-called dependency on modern medicines is the reason for its undeniable popularity and acceptance as a first-line treatment. Sadly, many people fall sick at an earlier age and crawl across their lives with the burden of their health issues.

Anyway, developments of modern medicines could be marked as important milestones in human history. The attempt showed the scientific prowess of human beings.

Many of the attempts had a social aim too. For that very reason, vaccines didn't offer money-making opportunities in the past. By the 1980s, vaccine makers became financially sick. Some analysis also pointed out how the industry thrived on the fear of people in third-world economies. Of late, people question the quality of treatment delivered by the system and the depleting quality of talent.

Medical scientists around the world maintain disparities in their approaches to almost every case, which is popular each time. Covid-19 itself is the best example. Since the outbreak of the pandemic, the WHO and many medical scientists kept changing their opinion on the nature of the disease. Regulators kept changing treatment protocols. While millions have been hit badly, millions have been saved too. Initially, it was said aged ones and patients with comorbidities were more vulnerable. The mortality rate among them was more. But there were cases of octogenarians recovering and young ones succumbing to the virus's impact. There are cases of older ones showing resistance to the transmission and younger one's inability to resist.

The uncertainty of mistakes was branded as trials. The finding was that a half-dose followed by a full dose led to even higher efficacy, around 90 percent, compared to the standard dose protocol. It was quickly brought to light that this half-dose protocol was a mistake, and not an intentional plan. Nevertheless, this finding could potentially change how we think about administering this medication in the future.

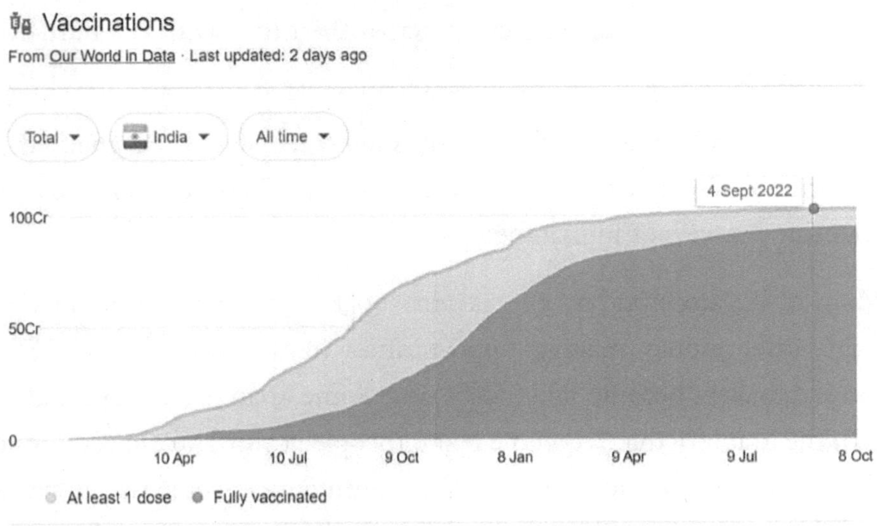

At one end where the authorities boast of having successful vaccination drives, the medical fraternity continued to experiment on humans.

Mene Pangalos, an executive at AstraZeneca working on the research programme, called the error a 'useful mistake.' The company didn't initially disclose that the half-dose cohort was a mistake, but Pangalos said that the error was quickly incorporated into the trial as an alternative dosing experiment.

"It wasn't putting anyone in danger," Pangalos said to the New York Times. "It was a dosing error. Everyone was moving very fast. We corrected the mistake and continued with the study, with no changes to the study, and agreed with the regulator to include those patients in the analysis of the study as well."

Scientists have no standard reason to offer how this disparity challenges their own earlier arguments. In the second wave, many young people with no known health issues succumbed to the infection, shocking even doctors. What's more, many young doctors also died of the infection.

Seven months after the breakout of the pandemic, scientists found Covid-19 was airborne, besides being a human-to-human transmission. A week earlier to it, WHO added new symptoms of Covid-19. By that time half a million people had died and over a million people became infected, mostly in the countries which boasted of having excellent healthcare systems. This showed either an inability of the so-called expert's insight to understand the nature of the virus or absurd claims of sophistication and great achievements in medical science.

Over many months several findings have been unearthed. Many of the findings were contradictory to the earlier findings. Still, people believe science speaks only the truth. Yes, science talks only about the truth. If a scientific standard keeps changing, it is either because of an unscientific element in it or because of a lack of wisdom in factoring in the changing nature of the human body. This also shows scientists have failed to read the virus's ability to make a change in the human body at different times. Let us not forget, centuries ago traditional medicines used to be administered for treating all the diseases which modern medicines treat nowadays. They used to treat patients to be resistant through immunisations rather than treating the disease to bring it under control. There was no regulatory system in place in those days and fraud found no place in the system.

We must compare the last 5 years of death rate in the same months and the reason too, to understand the truth. How many died last year at the same time with fever and malaria, dengue, pulmonary diseases/ infections, polluted environment etc.? How many people got killed in accidents, natural calamities and so on? During the lockdown period, people were frightened even inside their homes. Tagging a person as untouchable and isolating them was a trauma one underwent in the lockdown. Health workers coming along with an ambulance, vacating the room and premises, and putting people in quarantine centres were the dramatic episodes that killed a person mentally first, and that was more dangerous than Covid-19 itself.

What is the logic in quarantining the near and dear ones if a person gets positive? Modern medicine claims that there is no medicine for Covid-19. But the system wanted a positive-tested person to be in their hospital bed with apparently no or minute symptoms, to administer some medicines. As a layman, if you ask, what medicine they are using, you may not get a satisfactory answer. There are serious patients also along with less serious asymptomatic patients. While some die in the course of treatment, some patients come out with a half-life. No one ever questioned why an untreatable patient is taken on a ventilator if the chance of survival is bleak. The practice of taking people to hospital or even for quarantine was only a farce, as humorous as the treatment procedure. Once a patient was in the law regulator's custody, no one could do anything as it was a mandate to be quarantined according to the system. Thanks to the enforcement of social distancing. Neither could they shift to any other hospital for better treatment nor take any other remedial measure. The worst part was all the near and dear ones were denied permission to see or console the infected. The saddest thing was many of the Covid-19 tagged people succumbed to death deprived of their last rites, and seeing their people one last time, left a deep regret or wound in the minds of their dear ones.

Chapter 18

How Well Medical Science Could Save Humanity

Advanced countries developed many medicines that would last centuries, by pumping in huge capital. While the unquestionable drug delivery made many patients sicker, only a few were lucky enough to be the beneficiary of the wisdom. Many countries, including India, banned a large number of drugs of the last century after using them on patients of misfortune.

We believe harnessing the strength of science is essential for saving humanity and better living by exploring new space through human intelligence. Its business connotation, however, cannot be kept aside. Science cannot sustain as long as scientists are paid hugely for their job, besides the huge profit on the capital deployed on a scientific project.

When there is a capital intervention in the development of science, especially in life science, the end-receiver can be the victim of future failure or beneficiary of the wisdom. As far as life science is concerned, going by history, new developments have killed, maybe an equal number of people, as much the medicines saved. There are medicines which can accelerate a patient's death after a temporary period of recovery. The irony is that where a particular drug is saving lives, it can also be responsible for the rising deaths by drug resistance.

In India, more than 440 drugs have been banned, after using them for many years. In Europe and the United States, the list of banned drugs may be longer. Incidentally, most of those banned drugs had first originated in Europe and the U.S. by virtue of their discoveries in the same geography. If we argue that modern life science has killed more people, as mentioned in earlier pages, it might be termed insensible, but something that is an undeniable truth. We predetermine that there is nothing above the term called science, that is ultimate, and we do not have any dispute about it. But the fact is we are calling business development science. Every research happening in medical science is only a business development initiative since medical science has become a life-saving business. This business is worth trillions of dollars. While the developing nations contribute to it by way of bacterial and virus infection, malnutrition, the developed world contributes by way of lifestyle diseases. Both the segments, one way or the other, keep it booming.

Does anyone have an estimate of deaths related to drug-induced morbidities and early deaths? Most of the death, taking place in hospitals world over, are the result of drug failure or doctor's wrong judgement. We are aware that science cannot prevent the phenomenon of death, and it may just help lengthen the time of life in certain cases. But many patients either die early or succumb to leading an under-quality life due to modern drug administration. People who suffer from some types of cancers, which are asymptomatic at an early stage, are seen to become bedridden since the day the treatment of chemotherapy, radiation therapy, or immunotherapy begins. That effectively cuts down their life.

There are many other patients while carrying their pain during the course of their treatment, who find relief from traditional and herbal solutions. There are instances of patients, who lost all hopes after being on expensive drugs for long and returned to a near-normal life after opting natural remedies. How miserably modern science has led to the reduction in quality of life in their cases is a matter that we must ponder.

Looking at many cases, it seems modern medicine was groping in the dark, as it couldn't make a stable profile of the worst pandemic of 2 centuries, despite many boastful achievements. The fact is having used these traditional medicines, until you live, you live a life without agony.

Covid-19 pandemic is the finest example of modern medicines gone wrong. Most of those who were on modern medicine for treatment suffered other health complications. The pandemic alone is sufficient to justify the argument against modern medicines. The death of a number of highly talented doctors also showed modern drugs are more dangerous than natural remedies. This was evident 3 months after the pandemic broke out in India, when people began to use home remedies and Ayurvedic solutions. Much before the government released a protocol for Covid-19 management through Ayurvedic medicines in asymptomatic and mild cases, people were using the medicines as their individual options. These people developed no post-recovery side effects. At the same time, those who used modern medicines suffered serious side effects soon after their recovery.

Nora Foulkes, 87-year-old suffered from hypothyroidism, but her routine treatment was stopped when she contracted Covid in December 2020. She died from cardiorespiratory failure in April 2021 at Glan Clwyd Hospital, a post-mortem examination revealed. Failure to restart the drug when she returned to her care home contributed to her death.

All the previous pandemics also almost disappeared in their natural course before an effective medicine against it came into existence. The best example was the Spanish Flu that disappeared in 2 years without the support of vaccines and targeted medicine. Even in the case of the Covid-19 pandemic, many countries, especially in Asia and Africa, where the mortality rate was lower than that of the U.S. and Europe, used their traditional medicines. Failure in rightly profiling the complete nature of virus infection, modes of its communicability, the mystery of origin, etc., were not constant. Scientists had the variable interpretation. Almost every day we used to hear new findings of scientists about the nature of the coronavirus. None of the findings were consistent.

People did not know who was correct and what the truth was. Not even scientists could say when researchers had different opinions about the virus whose findings were correct. Every time, a new version of the argument came up. Media used to carry it as hot news.

This is an open letter of 32 doctors and health experts from across India, Canada, and the U.S. who appealed to the Centre, State governments, the Indian Medical Association, and medical professionals to discourage the use of medications and diagnostics that have no supporting evidence for the treatment of Covid-19.

While there continues to be much uncertainty amidst the outbreak of this novel disease, there is now substantive high-quality scientific literature that provides unequivocal guidance on the clinical management of Covid-19. Despite the weight of this evidence and the crushing death toll of the delta wave, we find the mistakes of the 2021 response being repeated in 2022, the doctors wrote in the letter.

These mistakes include prescribing medications like vitamin combinations, azithromycin, doxycycline, hydroxychloroquine, favipiravir, and ivermectin, that are backed by limited evidence that they are effective against Covid-19.

"Such wanton use of drugs is not without harm as the Delta wave has shown. Outbreaks of opportunistic fungal infections like mucormycosis in India and aspergillosis in Brazil were attributed to the widespread abuse of inappropriate medications," the letter reads.

Even today, the origin of the virus couldn't be ascertained. The prognosis remained mysterious. The world deliberately opted to stop an investigation, after the pandemic. It was good for some, though a vast majority of people who had no influential voice suffered inexplicably worse. No one was subsequently interested in knowing whether the virus emerged from cranes or other birds, or from the laboratory of Wuhan. In May 2020, Spain had killed one lakh minks in a farm in Aragon after finding the mammals were carrying coronavirus.

As Scientific Reports said in October, 'a significant number of mammals could be susceptible' to the virus. This would question the effectiveness of a possible vaccine, as animals would continue to carry the virus. Illness is not a crime. Any being, be it animal or human, born on earth can have an illness, may carry bacteria and viruses. Apparently, science killed more human beings, because of modern medicine misuse at multiple levels, inadvertently because of highly influential capitalist's businesses and the ruler's (rulers of all times) lust for power. Science, especially life science, needs a reinterpretation, since what we call science lacks wisdom, as it has generated more serious reactions than giving proactive or positive results. There could be no better examples of the mismanagement at the Covid-19 situation that led to the death of over a million people and sickness of several more.

Chapter 19

Drug Business Thrives on Fabricated Fear

Fear is a state of mind with a bearing on one's living circumstances. People who have no option but to work in a hostile situation during a pandemic have to live in fear for a long time, even when they don't want to. But those who have enough resources to live locked and safe can afford to live in fear of the pandemic much longer. The 21st-century pandemic has brought out one thing much more vividly; no one can live for long with the fear of infection, being locked inside. Eventually, and sooner, the fear has to be set aside and face what nature rewards.

There was a conundrum around the severity of the coronavirus. Media reports, discussions, videos, texts, and all modes of media presented it as a deadly terrifying disease. Clinical researchers, virologists, practitioners of traditional medicines, Nattu Vaidyans, and even political leaders did not spare a chance to chip in their comments, raising people's apprehension of the disease. People were so fearful that a Covid-19 patient living in the neighbourhood was seen as a ghost. The media had such an impact on people that they did not question the harmfulness of Covid-19. It was indeed contagious, as the number of infections was reported in clusters. People were terrified, as they were apprehensive; their questions were unanswered, and they were seeing this as an inappropriate way of managing the situation. As months passed, and medical teams started foraying their bit to control the situation, the fear was replaced with hope, but how far?

The situation was, anyone could frighten the masses, showing the unexpected people scenario, their helplessness, and a big number of death tolls. People in high rises stayed put for months together as they could afford to sustain themselves without moving out. But those who were compelled to work as soon as their pockets dried out, subsequently realised that the pandemic was a passing thing. They challenged the virulence of the virus. There were even those who were working and travelling throughout the lockdown and were never infected.

The rising death tolls touched hundreds, thousands, and then lakhs, and it was enough to instil the fear that this was something big and uncontrollable. People who had no option but to work and meet ends had to foray out despite the severeness and lethality of the virus. They could not afford fear, for it was a question of survival. The ones who could afford to stay indoors could well afford to foster fear too. This fear was after all only a concern of convenience. However, what made Covid-19 more terrifying is the fear and uncertainty it instilled in people for the virus.

The existing and yet-to-be-eradicated infectious diseases like tuberculosis and malaria continue to kill people. The daily death toll numbers for these were seldom reported. But if the number of deaths by tuberculosis is reported daily against Covid-19, tuberculosis seems to have a larger impact on daily deaths and is an endless pandemic. But despite its prominence and impact, people are not afraid of Tuberculosis because medicines are established, and the disease is not presented so aggressively in mass media as Covid-19 is.

Every day thousands die in every country as thousands are born. In normal circumstances, death is not counted, and so the death toll on normal days cannot be compared with the death toll during the so-called pandemic. My study has convinced me that the counting of the death toll has made the pandemic more horrendous than it was.

And in all this buzz and fear, what seems to be silently creating a storm is the medical and healthcare industry. A lot has been churning from bringing uncertainty to certainty on the Covid-19 diagnosis and treatment scenario. The fear has been brilliantly cultivated to sell some failed drugs and drugs of other targets, which were reassigned to develop vaccines. The business from vaccine sales has been worth trillions, although the long-term result of the vaccine is still questionable. The strategy for selling the vaccines was a wolf cry, followed by the introduction of the vaccine.

The BBC recently questioned a dealer who was offering what appeared to be fake remdesivir on the black market. The dealer claimed that the drug was '100% original,' but the packaging was full of spelling errors and the firm manufacturing it wasn't on the list of companies licensed to produce it in India. The dealer shrugged and asked the BBC reporter to get the drug tested in any laboratory and that the firm had no presence on the internet.

The anti-Covid-19 vaccine came up at a spectacularly magical speed, one-tenth of the normal time, negating all the wisdom of science, and the much talked-about clinical efficacy. In hindsight, everything appears an utter sham, a serious trade based on the fear created in the panic-stricken community. Rightly plugged from all sides, people's doubts have no space for an answer.

Let's see this example. Herbivores used to graze together in jungles, often in large flocks. Out of thousands, some never return from grazing, having faced their ultimate natural fate. The animals may or may not be aware of their fates, and they cannot express it as human beings understand. They work on instincts and may or may not be able to avoid predator attacks on them. But they never stop their routine grazing. The prey and predators are out for their food.

The prey does not opt for an alternate life, either they don't know of one or are helpless. In fact, they choose to live in an ecosystem that is shared with their predator.

On the other side, carnivores have no dearth of prey and also kill their contemporaries in the course of dominating their geography. In fact, the carnivores, which virtually rule the jungles of herbivores, also have enemies among them. Animals catch hold of their prey using their claws and teeth as nature armed them for their living and are capable of overpowering even more powerful predators than themselves.

I am not against any wisdom that saves the planet and mankind. If science holds up any wisdom, no one with a sane mind can either doubt its intention or question its findings. I do not doubt the strength of science.

In the Covid-19 scenario, science is framed as a carnivore, treating innocent humans as predators, and thus it appears that the humans are taken as civilised Guinea pigs. And this is the concern the world will have, perhaps once the pandemic fades away. We can only pray that the Covid-19 vaccine is no mishap of the future, under the various existing reports of post-recovery health challenges amongst Covid-19 victims.

In the modern world, human beings have become an object in all clinical science trials. We are made to believe that every clinical research and development is for saving humankind. But rarely has the result been so. As we watch certain developments and connect the loose lines of news appearing in the media, our suspicion becomes more reasonable and sensible.

We saw the pandemic spread like wildfire around the globe and even trigger brisk activities in clinical labs around the world in the spring and summer of 2020. Virologists and clinical scientists worked hard and burned their midnight oil to find something unique to steal the media limelight. Each day something new appeared in the media and one source negated the other. The alerts of the World Health Organisation (WHO) in early January 2020, after China reported its Wuhan misery, woke up every country and their respective healthcare regulators.

Simultaneously, fuelled by hefty public relations backgrounds, the global pharmaceutical giants became more active in their labs and dominantly took to the media with their ideas for tackling the medical challenges. The pharmaceutical giants in the world had built the clout to regulate the regulators. Armed with authoritative knowledge of the medical industry and healthcare challenges, pharmaceutical giants had become super regulators. No regulator in any country was able to negate what these drug giants dictated and claimed. Doctors blindly believed what the drug makers said and acted upon what the medicine sellers advised.

The patients and the general public hardly doubt their doctors, and thus it is easy to create panic among people. Interestingly in the Covid-19 scenario, modern medicine had taken the parenting responsibility for the pandemic. But the fact is, there was not just modern medicine but other forms of medicine. Modern healthcare technologies seem to be hand-in-hand with modern medicine streams only. Did they take birth together or can they be operated only in an integrated format? Why can't they be utilised for any stream of medicine? Or maybe in the course of time, the technologies evolved have been adapted the way modern medicine wants them to be.

When the panic button of the pandemic was switched on, the pharmaceutical giants found their business operations widening. Many of the medicines which were sold for mitigating the intensity of the infection could only prove severely counter-productive, with worst post-recovery complications or multiple complications in many people. Even savable cases succumbed to them, a fact that our healthcare regulators and doctors may not admit. Stocks of medicines were repurposed, and healthcare regulators were made to believe what these pharmaceutical giants claimed without any clinical database.

Doctors are not pharmacologists. They write what is introduced to them by the medicine manufacturers. But in the Covid-19 scenario, the panic-stricken world, something was better than nothing. Any medicine prescribed to them was taken with hope. Drug giants made use of this social fear syndrome and the human psyche. Most of the patients who died of Covid-19 were those who were treated with medicines, which were later removed from the Covid-19 treatment protocol itself. Hundreds of such lies stand sentries to the truth.

In the later part of this book, you may see some specific examples of certain drugs being first allowed and later withdrawn, making many patients victims of failed medications and decisions, making them the civilised guinea pigs under the veil of the pandemic.

The demand escalation of these vaccines only required a wolf cry. Once more fear was induced, and people rushed to take vaccines. Naturally, the panic-stricken humans found an element of elixir, even in poison. And who would question these multinationals who were making trillions worth of business supported by media, government, and regulators? Pharmaceutical giants, after all, have an additional edge for having a command of a community health system.

When a Mumbai Resident in Thane was in search of 3 vials of Remdesivir for a relative who was in critical condition in the hospital, he had a difficult time finding a pharmacy with stock, and it took him nearly 6 hours. The marked retail price for the medication was Rs 1,800, but the man behind the counter quoted a price of Rs 22,000 for the vial. The Mumbai resident was distraught and returned to his apartment.

His hope soared when a neighbour replied to an appeal he had posted on their residential society's WhatsApp group. The neighbour offered him 3 spare vials of Remdesivir recalling he had bought 8 vials of Remdesivir at a premium price to treat his father. Five vials sufficed, so as thanksgiving, he offered the rest of the vials at the marked price, not thinking of his financial loss.

Healthcare regulators and drug administration officials were aligned to not question any data given by drug makers, for the clout these healthcare giants had built. The government, regulators, and doctors were already abiding by what the drug makers claimed. They may not question the effectiveness of the vaccines which had taken virtually a premature offering. In the race for being the first one to introduce the vaccine, they knew the world was anxiously waiting, and many vaccine makers resorted to shortcuts. The longer the wait for the vaccine, the less will be the interest of the public.

After all, people around the world had begun to realise that Covid-19 is not as life-threatening as the scenario was created. So, a fast antidote was imperative to alleviate public fear.

Another realisation was if the people were paying for the vaccines, the makers may not meet their investments. All they needed was a bulk engagement. Many other vaccines were taking the market and not all vaccine makers would make it in time. The early birds approached governments of highly populated countries like India, which reported a larger number of Covid-19 cases, to sign bulk deals. No doubt, the influential giants had been ahead of more than 170 other candidates without letting anyone question how they could pull it off so swiftly. Additionally, there were surveys which stated the percentage of the population interested in Covid vaccines is reducing day by day, and that made these vaccine makers act more swiftly.

It is astonishing that in the case of the anti-corona vaccine, regulators had picked up feedback thrown by media reports instead of waiting for authorised data to come up with the application for approval. – How can we assure this statement? The reason would have been an urgency for approval to contain the pandemic. The world was waiting for a cure, and the vaccine makers knew the regulators would not raise even a genuine doubt. As public fear and the hype about the virus started ebbing, the vaccine makers hastened to launch it before the vaccine became irrelevant. Off late, Covid-19 is seen as only a common cold but with faster communicability. However, the wolf cry, as in the case of diabetes, succeeded in opening a market worth trillions. India has the second-largest diabetes count in the world. Apparently, it is not the skill and stake of any drug maker, but how the drugs were marketed, and the standard of tolerance set, that made these drugs unstoppable. We must remember, drug companies sold trillions worth of anti-diabetes and BP drugs in India, trapping millions of Indians in the net of lifetime drugs. Today, foreign brands dominate more than 80 per cent of the insulin market in India. They achieved this by setting standard parameters for all people globally irrespective of ethnicity, race, or gender.

Now, with Covid-19, they have tried to rebuild a market that they found depleting due to public awareness about diabetes and blood pressure (BP). This fraternity is unimaginably and unpredictably cunning. The government and health officials are least bothered about the impact on people's long-term life; after all, they too are beneficiaries.

More than 170 vaccines are at various stages of development. The big 3, leading in the pack, have claimed almost completion of the process for emergency approval. Vaccine development typically takes many years before establishing its efficacy. WHO never expected the vaccine trial to be over so quickly. It projected the timeline for public availability only late in 2021. But the clinical trial of the anti-corona vaccine took only 7 months to complete and claim success. It was a race against time to reach the finishing point. The first phase of the trial began in April 2020, when no one even knew when the pre-trial development works started. By early December 2020, the vaccine was ready for the first inoculation for the public in the UK. The fallouts reported in the course of the trial were swallowed by those who reported them, as the trials resumed soon after the pause.

In October 2020, the American pharmaceutical giant, Johnson & Johnson, had to pause its vaccine trial after one of its participants fell sick. After this, the company suspended recruitment for phase 3 trials. The company did not share details of the sick participant, keeping the world guessing about a foul, which again may or may not be serious. In the previous month, the trial of Oxford University-AstraZeneca for its vaccine also had one of its participants falling sick, which was also unexplained. The participant was reported to have transverse myelitis, an inflammatory syndrome caused by viral infections. One of the participants in India also fell sick and eventually filed a case for compensation of Rs 5 crore after he found his nervous system collapsing after taking a shot. Serum Institute of India (SII), Oxford University-AstraZeneca's Indian partner and the world's largest vaccine maker, countered the complaint of the participant with a defamation case demanding Rs 100 crore. Earlier in April, AstraZeneca's trial had reported the sickness of a participant.

The high degree of PR heat on the vaccine launch has been interesting and simultaneously astonishing. The Covid-19 fear in a majorly hit country like India, where the maximum number of vaccines would be sold, had started waning. The 'Medical pledge' that 9 global pharma giants looked like a farce. The leading Covid-19 vaccine makers like Pfizer wanted its biggest market. It wanted a government guarantee of compensation for those who fall sick by its vaccine. It is questionable even how the U.S. Food and Drug Administration (FDA) was ready to approve before completing the third phase of clinical trials.

Many people believed the vaccine is not necessary because the terrifying Covid-19 is not life-threatening. It turns out that the danger is when an infected person is administered potentially dangerous untargeted medicines. Many Covid-19 patients had the misfortune of being subjected to untargeted medicines. Many patients might not even take the vaccine if it is sold for a hefty price, and thus vaccine makers took a defensive strategy by creating fear among people. After creating much fear about the infection, the government was involved in acting at large and projected as protecting their people from the pandemic, thus addressing their bulk sales challenge. Compelling the government to procure its vaccine at a 'decent' cost for public distribution either free or at a subsidised rate was a strategy adopted by medical giants who introduced vaccines early.

The level of fear created by those having vested interests now justifies the emergency approval sought by the winners of the vaccine race. Many others were yet competing to the finishing point. Eventually, as people acquired herd immunity, the unworkable vaccines were still administered, and it all sailed through for the pharmaceutical giants.

There have been a few reports of immunisation errors with Pfizer-BioNTech, Moderna, AstraZeneca, Janssen, Sinovac, Novavax, and other COVID-19 vaccines. In very rare instances, some people reported more serious adverse effects after getting vaccinated against COVID-19. But these were not thought to be caused by the vaccine. Children who were given the incorrect dose of a COVID-19 vaccine or who received a poorly prepared vaccine reported experiencing the usual side effects, like soreness at the injection site, a headache, and a fever.

According to the World Health Organisation's global database of individual case safety reports, 24% of all case safety reports in children after receiving COVID-19 vaccinations are related to immunisation errors. These errors can include administering an adult dose to children, using the vaccine on an inappropriate age group, underdosing or overdosing a patient, using unapproved COVID-19 vaccines, scheduling doses too close together or too far apart, preparing the vaccine incorrectly (such as omitting a diluent), administering a COVID-19 vaccine instead of another vaccine, and not adhering to proper storage conditions or using expired doses.

But what will be the reaction and complications after a year, even the vaccine markers and clinical scientists did not know. Only God and the vaccine makers may know how many human beings will pay for their life for satisfying themselves with the vaccine.

The scared victims took vaccines for a sense of peace, not knowing their fate as being the prey of medical science. Some might live longer, while others might have complications. The years ahead are crucial, and the world has to watch it.

It is necessary to understand if any of the anti-Covid-19 vaccine makers are getting ready with a solution for managing any probable complications of post-vaccination. Who knows, the aftereffects may become a bigger tragedy than the Covid-19 pandemic itself.

Chapter 20

Intimidating Toll-Count, a Needless Exercise

A pandemic becomes scarier when the death toll is accounted. This mathematical exercise creates only panic. Countries ruled by dictators never report the death toll caused by war, violence, and pandemic, but in a democracy, it is difficult to hold back the number. We need to understand the fact that in normal circumstances also every day, death happens. The aggregate number is hardly reported daily.

There is no doubt; the virus was used for intimidating people. Today, a common cold, fever, and cough due to climate change are suspected to be Covid-19. In a country like India with fast-cycling weather conditions, catching a cold, cough, and allergic sneeze are just common, which our old generation used to treat with home remedies. In the recent past, these could be Covid-19 symptoms. A Covid-19 victim is looked at with suspicion, and people keep distance from the infected person. Every viral fever is infectious, but isolation was never done before.

The test kits calibrated for diagnosing Covid-19 indicate positive for Covid-19, even in the case of a viral fever. And that is one huge challenge people were facing. But the hope for this trend was that people were tempted to treat such cases with home remedies, unlike the pre-Covid-19 days.

Earlier people used to visit a doctor immediately on catching a cold and running fever. Then an antibiotic dose followed for settling with the viral sickness. On average, a child under 12 years living in cities used to visit a doctor at least twice a year for viral fever or other infections. The authority did not count such cases. A person aged above 50 years starts visiting doctors on a regular basis for one or another health disorders. Deaths in hospitals are common. But no one kept a count of the deaths and reported it daily. Even if it was done, it was not broadcasted daily on the media.

Daily new confirmed COVID-19 deaths per million people, Dec 17, 2022
Our World in Data
7-day rolling average. Due to varying protocols and challenges in the attribution of the cause of death, the number of confirmed deaths may not accurately represent the true number of deaths caused by COVID-19.

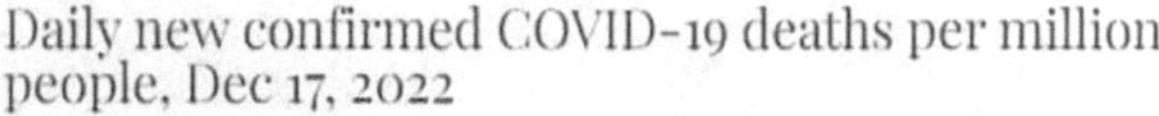

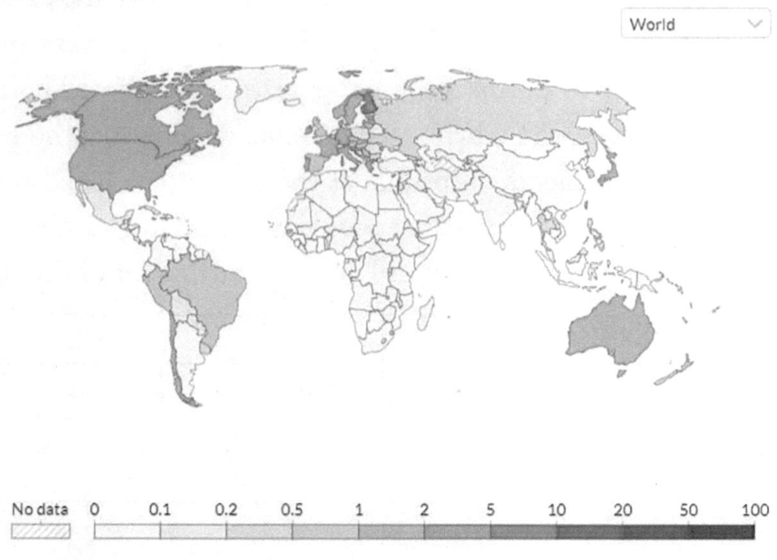

On average, an estimated 1.60 lakh people die in India every day. That is not a pandemic toll. In normal circumstances, also, patients die of various diseases, including viral infections, which may not have killed other patients with the same intensity and the same health parameters. Hospitalisation is required only if the ailment is severe with comorbidity, or if the patient requires life support. Covid-19 is not vastly different from other viral infections, except for the fact that we were excessively afraid of this, and our struggle against this disease was made more dreadful. It left a stigma on patients and the location they stay in. Even the respectable healthcare personnel were classified as untouchable when tested Covid-19 positive. As we failed in our lockdown strategy, we also failed miserably in the way we approached this disease.

The death happens in hospitals, at home, on railway tracks, on roads, due to calamities from our wanton activities, and in many other ways, including suicide. Every hospital mortuary is full every day. Normally, no one is bothered about such death toll other than the victims' relatives, friends, and closely known individuals. During the pandemic days, the death toll because of Covid-19 was counted every minute, while the number of deaths from other reasons was not. The toll of natural death during the Covid-19 pandemic was lower, although the socio-economic torments on people at the cost of the lockdown had been too rigorous. And how many people went missing or died due to the lockdown? The government did not have any count of the same.

India	
Total cases 4.46Cr	Deaths 5.29L
Worldwide	
Total cases 62.2Cr	Deaths 65.6L

The post-Covid-19 period reflects the severity of the lockdown consequences and the socio-economic troubles of pandemic mismanagement. I call the measures of pandemic management highly ruthless, mindless, and senseless not by one country, but by the world as a whole, including international organisations. The mismanagement was based on half-baked medical feedback, confusing research signals, wrong assumptions, presumptions, and the endless stream of image-building media features. This is the face of the modern world.

Excess mortality is a metric used by researchers to compare the number of expected deaths with the actual number of deaths during a time of upheaval, such as during wars, outbreaks of diseases, or natural disasters. Many scientists believe that this is the most reliable way to gauge the impact of a pandemic.

Data collected from more than 30 countries with estimates of excess deaths show that there were nearly 600,000 more deaths than what would be predicted in these nations from the onset of the pandemic to the end of July. Out of those 600,000 deaths, 413,041 were officially attributed to COVID-19.

The politicisation of the statistics became a way for countries to compete with one another, instead of working together to find a solution.

When deaths began creeping up in Europe, Lasse Vestergaard was one of the first to notice. Vestergaard, an epidemiologist at the Statens Serum Institute in Copenhagen, leads the European Mortality Monitoring Project (EuroMOMO), which aggregates weekly all-cause death data from 24 European countries or regions. Between March and April, EuroMOMO's tracker showed tens of thousands more deaths than expected — about 25% higher than the official COVID-19 deaths figure. Infections were slipping under the radar because of a lack of testing, and because different countries counted deaths in different ways — excluding deaths occurring in care homes, for instance. It was nearly impossible to get a true sense of how countries were faring.

So, researchers, journalists, and politicians focused on calculating excess deaths. Excess deaths are a metric that compares all deaths in a given week or month with the deaths that statisticians predicted would happen without a pandemic. This metric is useful because it doesn't get bogged down by cause. The prediction is usually made by averaging the number of deaths over the previous 5 years.

Birth is a reality, and death too is. When the Covid-19 stormed the world, every country began to count the death rate daily. But no one did ask how many people are dying on earth due to poverty, malnutrition, pollution-induced diseases like various types of cancers, or road accidents, death by drug overdose, drug resistance, and other lifestyle diseases. The number of deaths was rising fast and has always been much higher than what the pandemic reported. It is evident, every death accounted for in Covid-19 toll was not for the reasons of the virus alone.

Chapter 21

Mask Matters

A Times of India article on Thursday, 17th November 2022 states that "The Centre eased the mask rule during air travel which was in practice since the onset of the COVID pandemic. The Centre's decision comes at a time when cases of COVID continue to decrease in the country."

In Singapore and many other countries around the world, it's common for young children to wear masks against the Covid-19 norm. But aside from the protection they provide against the virus, do masks might pose a risk to children's long-term development?

There is no globally accepted consensus on this matter, but some experts believe that babies and children under 2 should not wear masks due to the risk of suffocation.

"The age limit for the use of masks by children is not yet a scientific definition," says Adamos Hadjipanayis, president of the European Academy of Paediatrics.

As facial expressions are a key component in human communication and child development, masking can hinder that process: "We learn emotions mostly through the face."

"Masks could potentially have a negative impact on children's language development. They look at the movement of the mouth and see the lips and tongue move. If you just think about the 'th' sound, the placement of the tongue is so important."

The Covid News Updates

- "The Kerala government on Wednesday brought back the face masks mandate in the state, in the wake of a surge in COVID-19 cases reported in many other parts of the country. It also announced that any violation would be punishable under the provisions of the Disaster Management Act and other relevant laws."
- "Amid fresh COVID-19 concerns in different parts of the country and apprehensions about a possible fourth wave of the pandemic, the Karnataka Government on Monday decided to issue guidelines making wearing face masks and maintaining social distancing compulsory."
- "Amid rising coronavirus cases in the country, wearing masks in crowded places could be made mandatory again in Maharashtra," state Health Minister Rajesh Tope said.
- "Masks are compulsory in Punjab now. The Health Secretary is issuing a detailed advisory for the people. Just remember to wear a mask when you step out of home for any emergency/ essentials."

This and other news made for the breaking news and headlines in the media as masks were made compulsory in public spaces.

The Mask Effect

Wearing masks and personal protective equipment (PPE) for extended periods can lead to physical and mental fatigue, as well as decreased work efficiency. Tasks that are performed while wearing masks take longer to complete and are less efficient than when no masks or PPE are worn. This is due in part to the fact that wearing masks and PPE can reduce the amount of time that a person can sustain an activity.

According to researchers, prolonged use of N95 and surgical masks has a variety of adverse physical effects, including headaches, difficulty breathing, skin problems such as acne and rashes, as well as cognitive impairments. Additionally, it can interfere with an individual's vision, communication skills, and sense of thermal equilibrium.

Masks that fit tightly around the face can cause a build-up of carbon dioxide (known as hypercapnia) which can lead to increased levels of respiratory activity.

A hot and humid environment in the facial region with a mask on can cause discomfort and even hyperthermia. This may slow down the performance of manual tasks and would also significantly affect motor skills. The moist environment and pressure from tight-fitting masks also block facial ducts leading to an increase in acne with prolonged mask usage.

Frequent mask usage can cause shearing and breakdown of the skin and bridge of the nose and cheekbones. Additionally, this could be due to wearing tight-fitting masks.

Some people may develop skin conditions such as urticaria or contact dermatitis from using PPE, as they may be sensitive or allergic to chemicals such as formaldehyde found in masks and other equipment.

Others may react to Thiuram, which is found in the ear loops of surgical masks. If you experience any irritation or discomfort while using PPE.

The first set of Covid guidelines said that the mask was necessary only for infected individuals, then it was made mandatory for everyone, and later it was made mandatory for individuals even at home. However, authorities made very diplomatic claims like –

"Wearing masks anyhow does not have any side effects or complications as such, thus it should be a decision of the individual from within to protect themselves, their families, and the nation in preventing the rise of yet another epidemic," says Dr Rajan Sharma, Past National President, Indian Medical Association.

UNICEF has been working closely with other United Nations organisations, governments, and industries to forecast demand, procure masks at an acceptable price and required quality, and ensure fair distribution, particularly to low- and middle-income countries. Since the start of the outbreak, UNICEF has sent 385 million surgical masks and 23.3 million N95 respirators and reached 134 countries.

GENERAL MOTORS TAKES TO MASS MASK PRODUCTION

The coronavirus (COVID-19) pandemic has created a critical shortage of face masks across the world. Our heroes are on the front lines of the crisis without the protection they need to keep themselves, their families, and the people they serve safe.

Thankfully, with the help of engineers, designers, buyers, and people in manufacturing, we were able to convert our Warren, Michigan facility to produce masks in less than 7 days. This means that more heroes on the front lines will have the protection they need to stay safe and continue doing their important work.

This facility is estimated to produce up to 50,000 marks per day, or 1.5 million each month.

A Face mask that detects respiratory viruses

Just when we became comfortable breathing with masks on, and it was time for the government to call off the mandatory use of masks, researchers have invented a face mask that can detect common respiratory viruses, such as influenza and COVID-19, that are suspended in the air as droplets or aerosols. The highly sensitive mask sends an alert to user's mobile devices within 10 minutes if it detects specific viruses in the air.

A team of researchers have developed a new N95 face mask that not only has the potential to reduce the spread of COVID-19 but also kill the SARS-CoV-2 virus upon contact. The mask could potentially be worn for longer periods, which would lead to less plastic waste as it wouldn't need to be replaced as frequently.

The process can be applied to already manufactured polypropylene filters, rather than necessitating the development of new ones. This is a huge breakthrough that has the potential to save countless lives and protect people from this deadly virus.

The user can wear an unaltered N95 mask along with another polypropylene layer with the antimicrobial polymer on top, according to the researchers.

"We are hopefully on the other side of the COVID pandemic, but this kind of technology will be increasingly important," said Zha.

A Covid museum

A recent article from the Times of India discusses the plans for a Covid-19 museum that would serve as a way to remember and commemorate the items, experiences, and moments during the pandemic. The face mask you made at home, your child's homeschool routine, the poem you wrote in lockdown, your video recordings of online meetings and other happy hours - all of these things have historical value and could soon become artefacts. This museum would be a way for future generations to understand what life was like during this time and how people coped with such a difficult situation.

The National Council of Social Museums is working with a team of curators, archivists, and museum employees across the country to collect and preserve elements from the current crisis for a largely crowdsourced Covid-19 exhibition. The exhibition will tell the story of how the country has coped with the pandemic.

Chapter 22

The Medical Oxygen Fiasco

On a fateful day in June 2021, alarms resounded throughout the ICU at Jaipur Golden Hospital at 9:45 p.m., jarring the dozens of patients hooked up to ventilators. Some thrashed their limbs while others cried out for help, their voices garbled as if they were being choked. The mechanics rushed to the maintenance room to see what was possibly wrong while the nurses frantically grabbed small plastic pumps to fill the lungs of critically ill patients by hand. That night, 21 coronavirus patients died in Jaipur Golden, a respected hospital in Delhi, due to a lack of medical oxygen. Shaista Nigar, the hospital's nursing superintendent said: "It was a total breakdown. Nobody can forget that night."

The district hospital in Bihar's Gopalganj district received 3 ventilators from the Centre in September last year as part of the government's response to the Covid pandemic. The government had procured 60,000 ventilators for nearly Rs 2,000 crore, and roughly 17,000 of them were dispatched to the states. The tragic incident at Gopalganj district hospital in April highlights the severe lack of preparedness of the nation's medical infrastructure for a raging pandemic. There was a massive shortage of beds, ICUs, ventilators, oxygen, and life-saving drugs.

Renowned Cardiologist Dr Devi Prasad Shetty, chairman and executive director of Narayana Health, said, "Beds don't treat patients—doctors do."

This shortage of manpower is putting lives at risk. To save lives, we need more doctors—and we need them now. India's response to Covid-19 was laxed by an inadequate number of medical staff—doctors, nurses, paramedics, and technicians. The country has 37.6 health workers for every 10,000 people while the WHO (World Health Organisation) benchmark is a minimum of 44.5.

In May 2021, India's hospitals were overwhelmed with COVID-19 patients. One of the biggest challenges was providing enough medical oxygen for the sickest patients, as demand rose tenfold.

The oxygen crisis in India led many observers to question the country's planning and preparedness for such a health emergency. This is especially concerning given that this was not the first time India has faced a shortage of medical oxygen during the current pandemic.

In September 2020, the country was already grappling with a similar situation as case numbers rapidly increased, and medical oxygen production failed to keep pace.

In response to this latest emergency, the Indian government, the UN, and other humanitarian organisations have taken a variety of actions.

In many states across the country, the health infrastructure that was built up during the first wave of the pandemic was dismantled once it was believed that the outbreak was over.

Last November when Covid cases in Delhi surged to over 8,500 per day, many of the patients who needed hospitalisation found it difficult to get a bed. Even the temporary additional facilities that were set up in June couldn't cope with the influx of patients.

The 4 temporary facilities included a 10,000-bed centre in Chhatarpur, run by the ITBP, with at least 1,000 oxygen beds. Similar but smaller facilities had been set up in Dhaula Kuan and at the Commonwealth Games Village.

But, in February, when daily cases dropped below 200, the Delhi government declared victory over Covid, and the 4 additional facilities were dismantled. Two months later as the second Covid wave struck, Delhi witnessed an unexpected shortage of hospital beds. The average daily number of cases peaked at over 25,000, and the city was lacking in medical oxygen. As a result, 2 of the major hospitals - Rajiv Gandhi Super Specialty Hospital and GTB Hospital - had to cut the number of Covid beds in half.

To meet the growing demand for oxygen, tankers were airlifted from other countries, tankers that usually carried liquid argon and nitrogen were converted to carry oxygen, and railways introduced special 'Oxygen Express' trains. Industrial oxygen that is usually used in steel plants was diverted to hospitals, and the procurement and distribution of oxygen concentrators were increased.

The UN focused on getting essential equipment like ventilators and oxygen-generating plants, as well as implementing other measures to reduce the rate of serious cases, speeding up the rollout of vaccination programmes, and improving testing facilities. The World Bank Group provided over $3 billion in support of India's efforts to combat the COVID-19 pandemic. As part of this, Bank projects at the national and state level were working with India to address critical gaps in its oxygen supply systems.

At the height of the second wave, the Bank Group worked in close collaboration with global suppliers to enable the fast purchase and delivery of 29,600 high-quality oxygen concentrators for the country. The bank also assisted with sourcing other oxygen-related commodities within India, such as oxygen cylinders. The bank partnered with the NGO PATH to provide targeted technical assistance to 4 states - Andhra Pradesh, Meghalaya, Uttarakhand, and West Bengal - to strengthen their oxygen systems and build capacities. It also supported the central government on key transport and logistics issues related to medical oxygen in India.

Despite all this, on April 27, the Supreme Court was given an affidavit from the Centre that showed a projected deficit of nearly 1,765 MT of oxygen per day in 6 states - Maharashtra, Gujarat, Madhya Pradesh, Uttar Pradesh, Delhi, and Tamil Nadu. A top medical professional termed the Centre's failure to arrange for advance supplies of oxygen as "Negligence of the highest order."

India's Covid black market

Item	Usual price	Black market price
Oxygen cylinder (50 litres)	$80	$660-1,330
Oxygen concentrator	$330-930	$2,000-2,660
Remdesivir drug (100mg)	$12-53	$330-1,000
Tocilizumab drug (400 mg)	$540	$2,000-4,000
Fabiflu drug (17 tablets)	$15	$66-133

Source: BBC

BBC

The Oxygen Cylinder Black Market

The Union health ministry was criticised for its failure to build a war reserve of medical oxygen. Late in 2021, the ministry announced that it would create a buffer stock of medical oxygen to last at least a month, but it could not manage to do so. On October 14, the ministry's Thiruvananthapuram-based PSU (public sector undertaking), HLL Lifecare, floated a global tender for the supply of 100,000 MT of medical oxygen.

The original order called for a staggered supply over the course of 90 days, with the first 15,000 MT shipment expected to arrive a month after the order was placed. There would be subsequent shipments every 10 days. Even if the order had only been placed by December, this would have allowed India to build up a stockpile by March 2021. This would have provided crucial breathing space both for the patients and producers in the short term.

Industry experts estimated that the government would have had to pay Rs 100 crore for the stockpile of liquid medical oxygen. This is because each MT costs Rs 11,000, without factoring in the cost of transport or oxygen tanks. An official from HLL stated that the tender was cancelled after bidders quoted a price that was higher than what the government was willing to pay. The ministry only realised the need for such a stockpile in mid-April when Covid-19 cases began spiking.

The scenes of relatives in India desperately trying to find oxygen supplies for hospitalised COVID-19 patients alerted the world to an acute, deadly problem. This was not, however, the first time that the country's hospitals had been hit by a shortage of life-saving gas. This raised the question of whether there will be enough supplies when the next major health crisis hits.

Chapter 23

A Disaster Called Virtual Classes

Have we lost our wisdom? Children were made to sit on a ticking time bomb called a cellphone during the pandemic, and the effects of that we come to face now and will see in the coming future.

Online schooling, private coaching, classes for competitive tests, fine arts learning, and hobby classes kept them busy under the influence of microwave radiation. While these effects were not considered, excessive use of cell phones disturbed children's sleep, brain activities, and mental health, and induced a potential threat of cancer by exposure to radiation. Children were tied down to their rooms during the pandemic, adding to their existing physical worries. It was ironic, while schools were only concerned about completing the syllabus, parents were acting oblivious to their children's use of cell phones for long hours.

Parents and academicians were not willing to sacrifice an academic year for their children, yet ready to expose them to cellphones, which they so strictly controlled so far.

We had lost our wisdom, while we were redefining the concept of education instead of making it a holistic talent development.

In 2019, after a fall of 12 percent, India's smartphone sales closed around $38 billion in 2021 with a 27% growth year on year. Indians bought 19,406 smartphones every hour in 2021 with a record sale of 16 crore smartphones!

India was the most potential market, thanks to the demographic advantage and growing necessities of children! The market reaped the Covid-19 advantage that made people connect with the rest of the world. To those segments it was forbidden until the lockdown, Covid-19 transformed it to be a necessity. An evil necessity.

Most Indian States had banned smartphone use by children in schools. In cases where online education was a norm even before Covid, the ill effects of smartphones were already seen. Several studies have shown that the use of smartphones by children has brought much physical and mental damage to them because of their excessive use and consequent addiction to them. And no addiction can easily decamp a victim. Deficiency of eyesight and other physical problems were said to be common for children using cell phones expressively. Various studies pointed out that frequent use of cell phones by children disturbed their sleep, adversely affected mental health, and curtailed their brain activities.

Besides causing many health challenges, the use of apps on phones and exposure to many forbidden things were slated to ruin the children in many ways. Cell phones are known to emit microwave radiation known as radiofrequency-electromagnetic radiation (RF-EMR). According to studies, such radiation led to cancer over a period of time. Doctors say cancer develops over 10 to 20 years after exposure to such radiation. Set aside the impact that may emerge many years after. Is there any immediate benefit of using cell phones so excessively? The answer is, "No."

The children who usually use cell phones excessively are also found to be academic under-performers and overall, less competent in meeting any intellectual tasks. However, many parents carry the wrong notion that their children become smart and intelligent by being experts in handling smartphones. However, studies point out differently.

All the studies, research, findings, analysis, and conclusions had now fumed out. The Covid-19 lockdown sanctified the sin of cell phone use by children. It has been made necessary. If misuse of cell phones led some children to suicide before Covid, is it less evil now? It is a question of misguidance vs sacrificing an academic year. Let's not forget, suicide among children was not known before smartphones came to them. Social scientists and child psychologists are silent now and figuring out ways to bring a solution to this issue.

Schools had gone online, and classrooms used higher technology to make education available to children even in these tough times. From nursery to post-graduation, classes were conducted online, which was a fashion of only the elite class until recently. Suddenly the cell phone became a no-sin device for children. It became more important than books and pencils. No one thought about the ill effects of handing a smartphone to children for a long time when it was rationed pre-Covid. The situation came to a pass as children's academic years could not be wasted, we were all following a herd mentality. No one could think of risking going against the herd and thinking about their child's health over education. Parents did not want their children to be left out of the race.

No doubt, schooling has greater importance. But wrong schooling will only become counter-productive. And we saw the ill effects of it. Children became so addicted to smartphones in the lockdown years that post-pandemic, it is a critical concern to keep them away from smartphones. Smartphones have become an integral part of their lives. And having rationed smartphone devices now has aggressive side effects.

We need to prioritise what is more important. Isn't their intellectual development, behaviour, and culture more important? Will the children completely fail in their life if they miss the syllabus of an academic year or 2? Losing a syllabus is not the concern of one child but of the children world over. When a child can compensate for his or her lost time, the impact of over-exposure to smartphones in a compelling situation can be avoided. Prevention is better than cure.

Children in metros and cities hadn't stepped out of their homes during the length of the pandemic. Their immobility again created a high-level of stress and various disturbances, which were then inexplicable. They had been living with smartphones and televisions within their locked doors as they could not move outside their apartments. The cell phones had tamed them.

Lectures and mock tests gave the children no time even to breathe. Everything was scheduled tightly side-by-side. Children listened to their classes while in bed or at the dining table. They were restless and put to run like a machine working in multiple shifts. The children living in an urban atmosphere were under greater stress, and hence at a greater risk. The consequences will only be apparent as we move ahead in time.

The online classes for primary-level children were senseless rituals with exaggerated importance. This ruined the small children, who should have been familiar with toys, instead of smartphones. On the other side, there were parents who had also been deeply disturbed by their children's addicted engagement with their phones. Nevertheless, they were helpless. Many a time, this created a rift between mature parents and adamant children. Finally, the parents were forced to budge and sacrifice their principle.

In all these trivia of the reformed education system and the undeniable pressure created, how could the economically poor people, who have more than one child, afford a smartphone and internet data cost? The lower income group could not afford the online schools under the pressure of job losses and cannot afford it, at least in the pandemic scenario.

Many parents, whose income was disturbed after the lockdown, found the mobile phone model of schooling a bit tougher. No school cut its tuition fees; they did not even have the burden of maintenance. Schools also made huge savings on their utility bill charges. They incurred no charge for extracurricular activities. Everyone charged as usual.

In June 2020, when Kerala schools began virtual classes, a Dalit daily wage earner's brilliant daughter from a village committed suicide because she had no smartphone at home to be online, while all her classmates began to attend the classes.

There were thousands of such children in India's thousands of villages with no privilege to have smartphones. There were thousands of villages in remote areas and the periphery of metros like Mumbai with no data connectivity.

The outbreak of Covid-19 made online schooling a necessity, which in turn highlighted the stark economic divide between different classes of students. Students in rural areas or other underprivileged students did not have smartphones or internet connections to keep up with online learning like their city-dwelling peers. This created a clear disadvantage for these students, who would fall behind in their studies as a result.

According to Save The Children Fund, the coronavirus pandemic has led to the 'biggest global education emergency of our lifetime.' Globally, lockdowns enforced to stop the virus' spread have put 91% of learners out of school. According to the Save The Children Fund report, 320 million students in India have been affected by online classes. This has been the biggest global education emergency of our lifetime, and the poorest and most marginalised children are at the highest risk of never returning to the classroom.

According to an India Today article, Haryana Education Minister Kanwar Pal said the government was aware of the difficulties being faced by the poor students besides those living in villages lacking internet connectivity.

"We have made arrangements for online classes for classes from 9th standard to 12th standard. We are planning to provide tablets to these students. The decision will be taken if the schools are ordered to be shut beyond July," said Kanwar Pal.

There were autistic and physically challenged children who were not able to use the online platforms. The online classes left out a large segment of underprivileged children.

Remote learning presented several challenges for students with disabilities, who often find it difficult to follow online school programmes. This left many students with disabilities behind, particularly those with intellectual disabilities. Furthermore, they have also been negatively affected by other aspects of closed schools, access to school meals, and engaging in play and sports with their peers.

In 2020, a survey conducted by Swabhiman, a community-based organisation advocating for the rights of persons with disabilities, found that approximately 43% of children with special needs across

India might drop out of school because of the challenges they face with learning online.

Although children with special needs missed classes, they retained their health. At the same time, their metro-living counterparts were vulnerable to too many social, mental, and physical disturbances. Addressing their future trepidation was not a small task but beyond anyone's guess.

They were simply sitting, or we made them sit on a devastating time bomb. The parents were compelled to give their children the forbidden gadget without enlightening them on what to do and what not. It was like opening a road for their ruination because children were easily susceptible to misguiding.

Chapter 24

What is the Generation Alpha Coping With?

If anyone asks me what the next biggest disaster may be, I will say that our next generation—Generation Alpha (born between 2010 – 2024)—is set to face challenges, I say doubtlessly, for their education. The system of virtual classes for as long as 2 years has shattered our children, who were otherwise also carrying the burden of syllabus overburden. The concern is squaring up.

Now, we have lost the meaning of education, as we have lost the meaning of Kalalayam. The erosion in the quality of learning has much to do with the prescription of the syllabus. It has made our education system imprudently more modern under the false impression that our children will grow up and achieve everything upon learning through sophisticated systems. Our children learn everything from printed texts, except how to live a worthy life. The online learning system offers hardly anything to learn. Like many parents, I too am confused. Yet, we are forcing our children to embark on this virtually and to betray themselves. On the other side, we become victims of the business interest of the modern education system. Some business tycoons played their bets right. Three segments such as education, pharma, and algorithms thrived on the pandemic, fear, and a lost sense of people.

India had been a model of the finest teaching systems in the world. Indian scriptures and epics are in the form of questions and answers. The Guru has been an immaculately great embodiment and the term Gurukul too emerged from this word. Guru and Gurukul (teacher and school respectively) are inseparable from ancient civilisations. In all these civilisations, parents, teachers, and gods were considered equal. From them, a child learns good lessons. We came a long way by universalising education and removing discrimination, which led to a grand universal elementary education different from the Gurukul system. Now if we talk about it again, it will become a controversial subject.

Under the Covid-19 lockdown scenario, children haven't met their friends for several months. In the urban centres, they are locked up within 4 walls to live a life under the round-the-clock sight of their parents. Not many parents are concerned about the prisoner-like life of their children. Very few parents are aware of the new generation's minds. Others treat their children with a traditional mindset, leading to a clash and conflict of opinion. It is sharply going up in the urban atmosphere, where children and parents have limitations, besides the limitations caused by the reckless lockdown. Children are locked by pandemic laws and parents, though safe from the infection.

With the COVID-19 pandemic came school closures worldwide, affecting nearly 1.95 billion children in 195 countries. E-learning was a convenient and viable alternative to traditional classroom teaching and learning methods during the lockdown.

The COVID-19 pandemic increased the demand for e-learning platforms worldwide, as children were instructed to attend classes online from their homes. Given the fact that the formation of higher-order functions takes place during childhood years, e-learning poses an adaptability risk for young brains. The brain's plasticity reflects how neural circuitry in young brains responds to digital learning.

Several studies have shown that exposure to multiple screens can lead to structural changes in the brain, including reduced volume of the cortex, reduced integrity of the white matter region, and decreased grey matter in prefrontal regions like the right frontal pole and anterior cingulate cortex. These alterations can then adversely affect attention skills, processing speed, verbal intelligence, and sustained attention.

Prolonged use of the internet and staring at computer screens for long periods has been shown to reduce the functional connectivity of regions around the temporal gyrus, which is responsible for long-term memory formation and retrieval of learned material. Additionally, overuse of the visual modality and exposure to bright lights from screens can cause adverse effects on the visual system.

The memory of university or college, usually known as Kalalayam in Malayalam, comes with excitement, perhaps the most exciting in your entire life. The reminiscence renders a smile. I am very sure, for many people, life on the campus was remarkably sweet. Kalalayam means a place or a platform to develop skills and taste for a subject at a young age for a bright future. It was also a place for politics, arts and sports, great fun and what not. It was the spring season in many people's lives. Simultaneously, a campus could nurture values, the right thoughts, and broader mindsets among youngsters. In that sense, the name Kalalayam is prudently meaningful.

I wish our children could return to their typical Kalalayam. They must know the actual meaning of education; we must let them grow up as they desire. We should re-educate them about what are the colours in life that we experienced. They deserve it. Education is not just what faculties are lecturing. It is much beyond textbooks. Education should not be within 4 walls but in an environment where children meet other children, learn, experience, fail, learn from failures, and succeed in learning new things every day.

The world has seen the largest mass quarantine to date, with countries like India, China, New Zealand, France, Italy, the UK, and Poland implementing nationwide lockdowns. As a result, the average screen time increased as we spent hours on electronic devices such as TV, laptops, tablets, or mobile phones for work, news, entertainment or to simply stay connected. Although technology has been a saviour in these uncertain times, it does have its disadvantages too. The increased use of screens caused people to become more irritable, impacting their circadian rhythms, which can lead to physical and mental health problems. People were constantly exposed to anxiety-inducing or distressing news (e.g., new cases and death tolls) on news channels and social media, which caused anxiety, stress, hopelessness, alienation, and sometimes depression. While it is important to follow the health advisories issued by medical bodies, some people are developing OCDs, which is making their existing anxieties worse.

As per the psychoanalytic perspective, Generation Alpha is likely to be affected more strongly than any other generation because it is witnessing the pandemic at a very impressionable age. Experiencing such drastic events during the formative years of one's life can shape people's behaviour, personalities, and worldviews in important ways.

The outbreak of the pandemic has forced governments worldwide to enforce lockdowns as a measure to prevent the spread of the virus. This, in turn, has resulted in many industries shutting down, limited transportation, and schools being closed. Although there are many concerning health and economic issues that have arisen from the lockdown, there has also been a positive impact on the environment. Major cities across the globe have experienced a significant decrease in pollution levels due to the reduced emission of pollutants during the lockdown period.

Chapter 25

The Social Animal's Social Distancing

May 05, 2020, Hindustan Times

According to the latest COVID news, "Only 50 people are allowed at weddings, 20 at funerals," says the government. The Union Health Ministry had earlier advised against large gatherings at funerals to avoid possible Covid-19 infection declared by Punya Salila Srivastava, joint secretary, the Ministry of Home Affairs (MHA) said at the government's daily briefing on Covid-19.

Lost Friendship and Closed Doors!

The pandemic changed human friendships and relationships. The term 'social animal' was redefined as the circumstance that compelled the most intelligent animal on earth to be self-centred in the name of precaution. The gap in relationships widened, and each of us was moving into seclusion under pressure.

The Greek philosopher and polymath, Aristotle, said; "Man is by nature a social animal." It was after the era of Aristotle; every pandemic was caused by human-to-human transmission that historians noted. The pandemic might have happened in the ancient days too, but without too wide a call for social distancing as we see now. The world was much larger at that time, unlike what we call today a village. As the world shrank, people could make more friends far away.

The 21st-century pandemic turned everything topsy-turvy. How the pandemic until the last century influenced human relations was not known to anyone. Nor did anyone know about any research by social scientists on a change in the equation of human relations after each pandemic. Whatever the result of that exploration was, the 21st-century pandemic was teaching us a big lesson about human relations. A lesson that will remain etched forever on our minds.

Owing to the high-level transmitting nature of the coronavirus, the pandemic called for a quarantine of infected people and social distancing for others, to stay safe from infection. It was through quarantine and social distancing that the deadly Spanish Flu, the previous pandemic, was said to have been brought under control after 2 years of havoc. When we blindly replicated the defensive model, we did not address the challenge of modern society. A century is too long a period to bring a change to any society.

We were taught to believe that the more we become secluded, the better our chances of being safe. For the social being called man, quarantine or lockdown are big tragedies as a self-exile, living within the 4 walls of homes. In the process, we assigned our relationship-building process to cutting-edge communication technology.

Our relationships shrunk from meeting to making calls and chatting. But these exercises had limitations, as we are self-regulated to make use of them only for a dedicated purpose. An average individual meets many people every day on his way, be it a morning walk or running to the workplace.

Nobody used to keep count of it. Familiar faces exchanged smiles and talked. It was unimaginable for anyone with a sound mind not to see anyone outside the home for many days. We were familiar with the story of Robinson Crusoe, who had been trapped on a desolate island and suffered the agony of loneliness. The pandemic had made each one live without any social touch. Neighbours were afraid of exchanging smiles. In urban places, many colleagues relocated to places where they felt safe. A good number of them vowed not to return, ending all their relations with the town where they once lived and hoped for.

The pandemic realigned people's relationships to the worst degree. Urban life underwent a radical change, but that is not something to boast about. In normal circumstances also, human relationships in the urban atmosphere were not something great to talk about. The pandemic further severed the relationship, thanks to the mantra of social distancing.

The sound of a neighbour's cough or sneeze made us panic or even angry. People were afraid of seeing their neighbours opening their doors. Exchanging smiles between neighbours was a fashion gone out of time. Many people in masks were gasping as if they had pulmonary disease. The world was moving to embrace a new equation as the pandemic continued to ravage mankind. Aristotle's social animal, the same species, was oddly practicing social distance.

In an open society like ours, people are naturally connected, warranting the term civilisation. On average, a person is known to have connections in one way or another with 100 to 150 people depending on his or her individuality. The pandemic has reduced this number, altering the social equation. At the same time, social media widened the scope of human connections, which will only ruin us further. The pandemic and our over-dependence on technology realigned our social relations, perhaps retracting us from our civilisation.

Chapter 26

The Omicron Variant

The world pressed the panic button against the pandemic when it started waning. However, a warning much before the first case of the new SARS-CoV-2 variant emerged was only an effort of exaggeration with a suspicious intention. The warning bell rang 2 days before the Indian SARS-CoV-2 Genomics Consortium confirmed the first 2 cases simultaneously in Karnataka.

There have been many variants of SARS-CoV-2 that appeared during the COVID-19 pandemic. Some were raging worldwide, while others were fading away quickly. The omicron variant overpowered previous variants in transmissibility but was less severe.

India's first case of the coronavirus variant XE was detected in Mumbai.

According to an article dated 6th April 2022, "The first case of 'XE,' a sub-variant of the Omicron variant of coronavirus in India has been detected in Mumbai," as per reports.

As per the survey, "Omicron variant was found in 228 out of 230 samples (99.13 per cent cases) from Mumbai," a civic health official said.

Also, with India's high vaccination rate, especially in the older age groups and across the population, even if a new variant emerges, it is unlikely to have the severe impact as was seen during the Delta variant, said World Health Organisation (WHO) Chief Scientist Dr Soumya Swaminathan to TOI, in the wake of the WHO's latest report informing of a new sub-variant XE.

The Omicron variant of the coronavirus was identified in 171 countries and became the dominant variant in many of them. The world was experiencing the highest daily new COVID-19 infections since the pandemic started. Alongside this, there was now a better understanding of the new variant and its spread. Omicron is 3 to 4 times more transmissible than the Delta variant. The majority of people infected with the Omicron virus remain asymptomatic, causing only mild disease in those who are fully vaccinated. The number of cases peaks in 2 to 3 weeks, then declines just as quickly.

When the Omicron variant was found, politicians started screaming, experts began giving free advice, and breaking news and stories flooded the media. For the news-starved media, it was a celebration time, but the ones who finally suffered were the commoners. They were struggling to meet both ends, with the sword of lockdown dangling over their head. We all knew who flourished in the pandemic – not the novel virus alone.

Modern medicine and pharma moguls know more about human psychology than they do about medicines. The Chief Executive Officer of Moderna went a step ahead with a statement that his company could develop a new vaccination against the Omicron variant. He also expressed doubt about the efficacy of the old vaccine against the new variant. Is it not a new variant-a new vaccine scenario?

It was not a new virus but a mutant of the old. Many old scientists mentioned it earlier. Once your action mutes the virus, when the pandemic peaks, there is the possibility of it breaking out in another variant. That was the story behind new variants, but none of us listened to them.

Drug companies ran their PR works before the drug was even ready. Then they launched it. The lockdown generated a parallel economy as the old economy remained locked. Restrictions followed by waves after waves were only experimentations. Believing a sham several times can make us only fools. Can one be a fool several times, or permanently?

There are 2 ways to control the pandemic. First, allow it to spread naturally. Its power will wane naturally and vanish over a period. Drug companies may not agree with this. Second, a vaccine is ideal only after the pandemic settles down so that people can be better immunised. But we were given the jab when the virus was active. At resistance, the virus changes its nature. That is the reason new variants of the virus emerged.

Europe was in a mess for Omicron. The U.S. too reported an alarming rise in this new virulent Covid-19 variant. Some African countries had reported big numbers, but hardly a worrisome picture. For Africans, poverty has been a larger worry. While there were several things for the rich countries to bother with. That is why media in the U.S., Europe, and even India celebrated the Omicron wave with news in larger print space.

The Telegraph website reported a story that is a scary and unpredictable event of people spreading the omicron scare.

Travellers staying at the Gatwick Sofitel, a quarantine hotel, experienced an absolute fiasco. The hotel reported an Omicron-infected guest gone missing, creating an environment of chaos and fear among the residing guests. Security went around frantically searching for the missing infected guest but without luck. To add to this chaos was a hotel fire alarm for evacuation, which led to guests huddling together in the lobby.

Chris Styles, 57, a customer who paid £3,700 and had arrived with his wife from Johannesburg, South Africa, said he was horrified looking at the absolute chaos.

If asked how well the vaccination protects a person from infection, the answer would be ambiguous. Eighty percent of Omicron victims were vaccinated people. Some people even took the so-called 3rd dose as a booster. As vaccination coverage expanded, Omicron also struck new numbers. And for what? Fully vaccinated people got entry into places where unvaccinated ones were forbidden, but the vaccinated people continued to die of the virus.

The Telegraph also shared strange instances of countries paying incentives to their citizens to get inoculated.

Slovakia offers cash to those over 60s to get vaccinated

Slovakia is to give cash handouts to people over 60 who get vaccinated against Covid or have their booster shot, as its government aims to spur inoculation rates lagging behind others in the European Union.

The Slovakian parliament approved the payments today, giving the go-ahead to a proposal by the government which had at first considered handing out vouchers for hotels or restaurants but opted instead for payouts.

Those receiving booster shots by mid-January will get 300 euros, while over-60s who sign up for the vaccine by that time are entitled to 200 euros.

Slovakia is not the first country to offer incentives to get vaccinated. In October, Switzerland offered free restaurant meals or cinema outings to citizens who persuaded their friends to get Covid jabs.

Chapter 27

Changing Compulsions of Life

When the globe has shrunk into a village, the so-called novel virus has its roads wide open to run. When the virus globalised, human beings went into confinement, renouncing all luxuries and remaining undercover.

Washington State in the U.S. is nearly 10,000 km away from the Covid-19 Chinese city of Wuhan across the Pacific Ocean. It was in the third week of January 2020 that the U.S. had its first Covid-19 victim, who had flown from Wuhan, the epicentre of the disease. Covid-19 further devastated New York, the financial capital of the world. The U.S. paid the heaviest price for the virus.

The UK is nearly 6,000 km away, and Italy is more than 8,600 km away from the Covid-19 source. Both rich countries have been shattered badly by the pandemic. Covid-19 devastated almost all top cities in the world, far from where it originated. The pandemic had its effects resulting in a crisis worldwide. The virus fear reached villages where even the drinking water connection had not reached. The virus got globalised beyond expectations.

Globalisation, in terms of pandemics, is the speed of infection that conquered the globe. The fanciful term otherwise is generally used to define business expansion, connecting various industries at different ends of the world.

Globalisation is a progeny of someone's dream of a wider industrialisation landscape. As the world talks about globalisation, countries fight to protect their borders, a big paradox. Is the concept of borders only applicable for fighting a war? After all, war too is a two-way business. For some, it is for political advantage, and for others, it opens business opportunities.

Even when the world passed through lockdowns, robots, engineers, and workers were vigorously active in weapon-building factories, while coffee shops were made to pull down their shutters. When countries tightly protect their geographies, globalisation becomes provincial, benefiting only business aristocrats to become richer. Worse, some of these so-called borders have badly divided ethnic identities, creating splits between hostile countries. India is one of the finest examples, and Arabs also face similar pain in West Asia. Promoters of globalisation have never considered the agony of divided ethnicity. When borders are drawn and the so-called advantages of globalisation are sought, we do not try to ascertain the social realms of divided ethnicity.

In terms of the economy, realistically, globalisation, which is said to have contributed to the growth of the GDP of some countries, has never brought any benefit to the poor and middle-class people of developing countries. Growth in GDP hardly matters to the underprivileged but heavily supports many corporations and business rulers' global dreams. However, a lion's portion suffered, and we still foolishly believe that it has given greater opportunities to people who are having bigger ambitions.

Developing countries were more keen to globalise their industries with a dream to tap potential around the globe. While we were heavily engaged in exploring the business potential worldwide through the process of globalisation, we overlooked the negative aspects of it. Let us not forget, every living being is created with the comfort of living in the environment in which it is born. Replantation and root canalling are either an experiment or mechanical refitting of the root with the support of inorganic manure. In such cases, the quality of life is sacrificed. Globalisation has made many regions vulnerable to undesirable changes. As change is constant, so is vulnerability. We have seen it all in the spread of the pandemic. In no civilised country are domestic movements of people and materials between provinces ever curtailed. The pandemic seemingly robbed away this freedom and contained living colonies.

Many locations had been sealed and barricaded in isolation for weeks together. People rediscovered their geographic borders when they tried to cross over to 'other' territories as they routinely used to do. Before the pandemic, no Indian citizen needed any work or travel permission to go anywhere in India. Many metropolitan citizens didn't even know their district borders. Many of them crossed city borders daily for their livelihood.

Until the pandemic hit, no one was bothered about their geographic boundaries. But during the pandemic, people became increasingly suspicious about people coming from other locations. In good times, people were commuting across continents for business and money. It is interesting to compare this strange restriction with the pre-pandemic global mobility of having breakfast in Dubai and dinner in Singapore. Worse during the pandemic was visiting one's old parents staying far away or returning to the native place, as that too required a 'Pass' and a 'quarantine test.'

Before, countries opened markets to all businesses, giving huge tax exemptions to boost their economy. When denizens of the same countries suffered from a pandemic, governments or corporate giants who gained from this globalisation stood unconcerned. Corporations and governments wouldn't have been so rich without globalisation, and yet this diverse outlook.

The privileged ones wouldn't have enjoyed the luxury they did until the pandemic halted everything, even the benefit of globalisation. Villages were turned into towns as villagers sold their agricultural lands to business tycoons for a dream. Agriculture fields were turned into townships. What was a luxury until a decade ago has now become an essential item. Globalisation has changed eating habits, living styles, and mindsets. Rice and roti have been replaced by pizza and noodles. The local touch is replaced by the global touch in food, dress, and lifestyle. Countries' border limitations did not bother them. The border was only a subject of war. People were happily living on what was available to them since time immemorial.

No life perished for want of any of the daily essentials in the past. This truth indicates human beings could live without globalisation, even in better conditions and fearlessly.

The hardest truth is, hadn't human beings run crazy for globalisation, the virus wouldn't have killed even a single creature outside Wuhan.

Amidst all this, technology played a vital role. In India, technology was used to monitor Covid cases. The Arogya Setu App, India's Covid-19 contact tracing app, despite fears over privacy, had been downloaded 100 million times within 6 weeks, according to the information technology ministry.

The use of Arogya Setu, which means 'bridge to health' in Sanskrit, was made mandatory for government and private sector employees. But users and experts in India and around the world found the app raising big data security concerns.

The app uses a phone's Bluetooth and location data and lets users know if they have been near a person with Covid-19 by scanning a database of known cases of infection.

This data collected from individual users is then shared with the government.

"If you've met someone in the last 2 weeks who has tested positive, the app calculates your risk of infection based on how recent it was and proximity, and recommends measures," Abhishek Singh, CEO of MyGov at India's IT ministry which built the app, told the BBC. "While your name and number won't be made public, the app does collect this information, as well as your gender, travel history, and whether you're a smoker."

Narendra Modi, the Prime Minister of India, has tweeted in support of the Aarogya Setu app, urging everyone to download it. The app has been made mandatory for citizens living in containment zones too, and later at airports and offices.

The app store's location data, which is a prime concern globally, requires constant access to the phone's Bluetooth, which experts say makes it invasive from a security and privacy viewpoint.

However, Mr Singh of MyGov said, "Your data is not going to be used for any other purpose. No third party has access to it."

Also, people can fill out the form incorrectly and the government cannot verify it, so the efficacy of the data is questionable.

During the pandemic days, everyone closed their borders with a prayer for achieving one goal, a region to live with no fear of the virus. Yet, human beings haven't closed their nasty work on toxic elements, i.e., building bombs to kill enemies. The eagles, nevertheless, continued to stare at their prey for a new run over the carcasses on which the virus had a feast. Covid-19 changed the definition of globalisation, as the world remained localised. There would be a new term for this in the context of technological development and its influence. A human being could reach any end of the world without physically being there and the efforts are on to remotely operate everything. Artificial intelligence and computer-driven robot operations open new possibilities for remote-controlled factory operations. By sitting in India, an industrialist can now operate a factory on the other side of the Atlantic. The Pandemic necessitated the functioning of work by sitting at home.

Chapter 28

When Covid-19 Becomes a Litmus Test

A debate on how well modern medicines have saved human beings may happen repeatedly and draw respect for it. Nevertheless, it is also equally important to open a debate on how well the influence of modern medicines has grown to leave behind an ever-alarmingly large number of patients. It is an undeniable fact that drug giants could thrive on the increasing sickness of people. One can simply understand this fact. I have discussed in the earlier part of this book that there hasn't been any count of deaths caused by drug reactions, drug overdose, and drug resistance. But the clout of modern medicine is ferociously huge, that even the boldest authority in the world cannot think of constituting a commission of inquiry into this medical genocide on patients. I am afraid the world is moving through a more dangerous period. With all our achievements in hand and our knowledge of resources available on the planet, if we fail to tackle the challenges that we face, we can foresee doomsday for human beings. The Covid-19 pandemic was just a litmus test.

Anthropologists believe human life has been in existence on earth for millions of years. Virus and bacteria too lived along, perhaps harmoniously, barring exceptions. In the primitive days, when medical science was driven by logic without needing the so-called clinical pieces of evidence, human beings lived longer years. While modern medical science might dispute its apparent attempt to justify its achievements.

Jeanne Clement, born in 1875 and died in 1997, proved a human being can live up to 122 years. Many living examples have proved human beings can live for more than 100 years. There are pictorial and sculptural shreds of evidence of human beings' longer life in the primitive and prehistoric days.

No historian, geologist, or genealogist could offer firm evidence of the average lifespan of human beings before modern medical science invaded traditional healthcare practice, other than playing a guessing game. To put it straight, no one knew how long human beings lived in the pre and post-historic periods because there was no data that estimated the age of human beings living in the earlier centuries. But portraits and sculptures which depicted the ancient civilisations showed human faces with wrinkles and frailties of old age. What the pictures and sculptures indicated was distorted with new interpretations in an apparent attempt to misinterpret the lower lifespan of people in earlier centuries.

While ageing researchers are still groping in the dark, some statisticians try to compare the lifespan of human beings living in the modern era with the lifespan of human beings who lived in earlier centuries on whom no data was ever recorded. Let us not forget, this planet had human lives for millions of years. There is no believable data that shows higher death rates due to disease and poor healthcare support available to them in those days, but by famine or by natural calamities.

We don't need to go far away. Each Indian will have many examples in their villages and ancestral homes to show how long our ancestors lived without any health complications. In the Indian context, we just need to recall the life of our older generations and ancestors. Many of them had never had modern medicine in their long life. They used to smoke and drink locally distilled or prepared intoxicants. Every household will have a story about their ancestors living up to 90 years or more. Many of them have a story of never going to a hospital. Most of them never had a blood test in their life. Most of them never had in their life the unpopular modern menace called diabetes. They used to work like machines, unimaginable by today's standards. Yet, they had a better quality of life despite inadequate food under colonial rulers. They hardly suffered any of the pandemics, barring isolated cases, which were treated by the more powerful herbal medicines popular, but with variability in different geographies. I haven't heard of them ever going to a medical check-up during their lifetime. They lived a happy life without restrictions on the food they used to like. Their energy and immunity levels were far better than their next generation, who began to visit doctors after the age of 25. The increasing size of the population after the age of 25 became chronically sick. The blame was put on a poor lifestyle. But the actual reason for making a person chronically sick was the wrong beginning of medication. A doctor's last word never lets anyone consider another opinion.

After all, everyone is afraid of bad health. Allopathy brandishes so big an impact that makes a patient refuse to seek an alternate opinion. Even if the patient takes another opinion from allopathy doctors, the view may be confusing.

An average person, if digs deep into the history of modern medicine, shall see that the so-called allopathy in the overall time clock of anthropology is aged only a fraction of a second. Its performance in the early years was not life-saving, but more life-threatening. Yet, it could expand its clout and ensure aggression on the deep-rooted traditional medicines, which were more popular in every Indian village until 3 decades ago. Even now its vulnerability to mortality is higher in the ways of side effects.

Traditional medicines could have done better service to human beings if they had aligned with the logic that traditional medicine maintains. The unavailability of a patent for traditional medicines posed a challenge for large drug companies, which were afraid of traditional medicine formulators eating their business away. Drugmakers having a keener interest in building their unchallengeable base did not want a curing solution that perpetually salvages a patient from his ill health. They want a patient to be repeatedly a patient so that the medicine business never slackens.

Modern medicines are built on the capital power that is swallowing human beings now, and the process is feared to continue. The pandemic is only a curtain-raiser. The hurried attempts at the vaccine and the strategies to make it acceptable to people by triggering waves are pointers to a more dangerous future.

Some doctors said the vaccine effect would last a year or 2 if no variants emerge. Genome sequencing reportedly identified new variants in more than a quarter of the samples studied. The story makes the picture clearer. New variants are emerging that reduce the guarantee of the vaccine impact. People will have to repeat the immunisation. It may be unimaginable, but it is going to be a devastating truth. Henceforth, the probability of lifetime immunisation cannot be ruled out, so long as immunisation is not salvaged from the business trap, which is incidentally impossible.

Until 2 centuries ago 'allopath' was considered highly derisive by traditional medicine, which later flourished heroically. To justify the term heroic medicine means largely because of capitalism and the reorientation of healthcare as a business. Yet, it couldn't stop deriving the logic that remained in traditional medicines. The best example is Diabetes Mellitus. Even the name itself is derived from 2 ancient civilisations – Greek and Latin. Before modern medicine could spread its clout, the human world had survived pandemics. In countries where there was a strong traditional medicine system, the pandemic did not kill much of the population. Much before the emergence of modern medicines, all the primitive civilisations, be it Babylonian, Egyptian, or Indian, had in their texts remedies for illness. For more than one and a half centuries, modern medicine tried to dismantle traditional medicines by seizing essential and individual powers. Almost all early-day modern medicines were later withdrawn, proving them unsafe after killing millions of people.

We need to remember a fact at this juncture as we see unlimited drug overdose in the name of Covid-19 treatment, to treat the drug overdose, there is another set of medicines. The chain of medicine after medicine goes on endlessly carrying with it the miseries of human beings. It is a vicious loop created in the name of healthcare.

The system of modern medicine gained popularity only in the last quarter of the twentieth century; or say in the last 3 or 4 decades. The early years saw many adventures and test failures. Still, modern medicines could swallow the space of all traditional medicines and build their prevalence. This kingdom subsequently grew into a position where it could control everything. Now modern medicine has taken over not only the logical traditional treatment methods, which treat patients rather than diseases, but also governments around the world.

The system of treatment was a part of every civilisation. The treatment system survived centuries after the downfall of most civilisations. Even now the systems are alive for the namesake but remain stained by the shadow of the aggressive allopathy called modern medicine. Allopathy conquered the world, say the human world, at an astonishing speed. Allopathy virtually means a fictional empire run by drug czars whose wings are fearfully wide and theirs are the last words about the treatment. Doctors, who cannot have a different say on any medicine sold by influential pharma companies, are merely executors of their plots and plans.

More astonishing is its dictating power and unquestionable influence over rulers of all continents. Modern medicine has acquired the power to decide how long a human being should live and how well each human being could be made its customer. Every seller likes to control the buyer's market. Drug companies like to control the patient's market. Their business prospects depend on more people becoming perennially sick with one or the other disorders. The entire human life on earth is under the clutch of these drug czars. Every day, more people become sick, and this means more people fall under these clutches every passing day. Even if a person can survive for a day without food, he cannot survive a day without medicine. We are yet to open our eyes and look for the reason for this sorry state. Who is profiting from this sorry state of human beings? Strange!

We cannot make the situation better. The mirage called modern medicine has trapped us so dangerously in its net that an escape is unthinkable with our limited ability to question any medical logic. The death rate is on the rise. Lifespan is reducing, though ageing researchers do their work only to help drug developers justify their business. The evidence-based treatment legacy of modern medicine, however, made more people perennially sick. Yet, the fact is unquestioned because of modern medicine's façade called research data and scientific evidence. However, no one tried to gather any scientific data on people who died untimely due to drug-induced diseases or wrong treatments. The covid-19 death rate is one of the best examples where most patients died because of the wrong use of medicines. We cannot expect any inquiry into the dead bodies and ascertain the chemistry that caused the death. The government of any country in the world will also have to remain helpless. Even proactive governments will have to remain content with the answers served by the monarchs of modern medicine. Ultimately, all evidence seekers will have to swallow the excuses that the medical fraternity offers.

In the early days of the pandemic, people thought allopathy was losing the battle. But it could soon retrieve its space more strongly or say aggressively. Half-done research works moved into re-profiling for the treatment of new anti-viral strains. Large drug companies could ship out their old stocks. All old stocks have been injected into the Covid-19 patients in rare opportunities that the drug makers got. They managed to procure emergency approvals, showing data that they submitted to the regulators of their home countries and sold many drugs for a killing price. Our regulators had no time to verify the data as the outcry for a solution from various quarters surfaced suddenly. Works for many vaccines also began briskly. The attempt for a therapeutic solution did not gain speed as global drug giants were sitting on huge unsold baggage, which they wanted to sell somehow.

As the process of vaccine development and testing gained speed, some leaders could procure emergency approval also for final trials in the name of emergency use. When the hesitancy rose, the second wave swept across the countries where more people were reluctant to go for the vaccination. As the Nobel Prize winner, Luc Montagnier, who is known for controversial statements, pointed out the truth, "Vaccination drive during the pandemic period was unheard of in human history. The western world is witnessing a highly aggressive anti-vaccine campaign that the mainline media used to neglect."

India's regulatory authority of medical research, the Indian Council of Medical Research (ICMR) said the latest more serious side effect, Mucormycosis also called black fungus, is caused by drug overdose. Who was responsible for this? There was a treatment protocol in place. Still, no one is found guilty! If someone suspects that this has been a ploy to create a market for medicines that had no market, can his conclusion be construed as wrong?

The medicine, Liposomal Amphotericin B for the treatment of black fungus is costlier reportedly between ₹5000 and ₹6000 and was sold at double the price. More companies were planning to launch this product. Many multinational drug czars were ready to retool their factories to make this, making us estimate how far the black fungus was going to proliferate.

A belligerent lobby lays a big shield against any questioning of the logic of modern drugs and the marketing strategy of drug czars. When the Indian yoga propagator and Ayurveda entrepreneur, Baba Ramdev spoke bluntly, for which there was a hue and cry against him.

According to a Hindustan Times article in Dec 2022, Patanjali, co-owned by Ramdev Baba, recently issued a spate of advertisements called 'Misconceptions spread by allopathy,' claiming chronic diseases like hypertension, blood sugar, thyroid, asthma, and incurable diseases like autoimmune disorders and heart blockages can be cured by yoga, Ayurveda and naturopathy.

The IMA has decided to complain to the Food and Drugs Administration (FDA).

This is not the first time that Ramdev has had a run in with the IMA. In 2021, during the second wave of the pandemic, the yoga guru reportedly questioned the efficacy of allopathy in treating Covid-19.

Reacting to the claim made by the advertisement, Dr Santosh Kadam, general secretary, IMA-Maharashtra, said, "It breaches medical ethics. In neither field of medicine can you advertise to seek patients. We strongly oppose this."

There is freedom for everyone to make a defamatory statement against Baba Ramdev for saying what he had said. But could anyone prove what Baba Ramdev said was wrong? When Baba said so, what made the so-called Indian Medical Association (IMA) feel so deeply hurt that compelled it to threaten him? Are they afraid of him? Why is IMA so concerned about the image of allopathy? Is IMA afraid of any backlash in the aftermath of so many deaths and reports of drug overdoses that make people sick for a lifetime in some cases? These questions are unanswered. Instead of threatening him with a libel suit, they should have answered him with evidence to prove whether the Baba was bluffing or speaking out the truth.

IMA has no locus standi to retain the name 'Medical' since it does not accommodate professionals from other streams of medicine. Its terrific disposition even challenges the government. Somewhere, there should be room for open debate. The debate should cover the truth behind the hurried vaccine development, and answers to the anti-vaccine campaigners' argument. There should be answers to so many deaths and alarming levels of sickness. And there should be someone answerable for all the crimes of death and sickness.

Will the government assign someone to judge who has been at fault? Who will open the door of debate is the final question. Let's retain our right to know the truth that can save humanity against the punishment kept in the laboratories of medical business. Let the pandemic be no longer a potential opportunity if anyone has made a business calculation. An attempt to save precious human life is admirable only when it has an undoubtedly humanitarian touch.

Chapter 29

All That Went By

This book is my revisit through the pandemic days as I witnessed the sights of the street and urban peripheries. Being in the field of Ayurveda, I was actively working during the entire tenure of lockdown and had to go around under emergency services. I behold all the pathetic memories of Covid-19 and I am bewildered and dismayed over how our medical science remained miserably confused, and how our policymakers through foul policies failed to manage the spread. I am extremely dejected over the misery of millions who lost their livelihood and life; we could have saved them. Every person who experienced the pandemic could have seen how a generation was overhauled at the cost of the vulnerable ones and sadly, the vulnerable ones constituted a majority of the demographic.

Behind the failure of medical science and policymakers, anyone with common sense could have circumstantially concluded that the pandemic was only a plot planned and executed by a section with a global blow, to which many countries knowingly or unknowingly fell victims. More appalling was to watch some shrewd players at every level from the local self-governing body in India to hospitals and drug companies, could cash in on the chance misery of the public.

Keeping fear intact was the interest of this fraternity and they succeeded. Medicines approved and disapproved, allowed, and later withdrawn, virologists' different versions of arguments about pathogenicity and yet the unconfirmed nature of the virus particle etc. showed only the defenselessness of modern medical science. Apparently, these might have been done in confusion, but with ulterior intentions.

The book unravels it while dwelling on the origin of the virus, pandemics historically turning into endemics, modern drugs' big claims, mysterious side effects, and confusion about modern medicines despite claims of many big achievements and breakthroughs. The world was put through chaos, and a lot of confusion. Constant policy changes in the government and local governing bodies added to the public confusion.

In India, from 3 January 2020 to 14 November 2022, there were 44,666,924 confirmed cases of COVID-19 with 530,532 deaths, reported to WHO, before even the second and the anticipated third waves were over. Such deaths are a testimony to medical failure because the nature of the disease was not firmly understood.

A pandemic a century ago was a bigger challenge than what it could be now as modern medical science is said to be far more advanced. Yet, Covid-19 shook the world. The world's most advanced country, the U.S. paid the heaviest price in terms of casualties. A country boastfully the most advanced in every sphere, failed in the Covid-19 ordeal.

The second and the third wave fear coincided with the launch of the vaccine, which was developed in so short a period as one-tenth of the average time required for vaccine development. Immunisation programmes in every country continued while the pandemic waves moved up and down. This was the first immunisation programme people approached with hesitance and suspicion about its workability and positive result. The second wave was a big blow in most places claiming lives heavily, and public hesitancy towards the vaccine vanished because the atmosphere was of immense fear.

Scientists had differing opinions about the nature of viruses, and medicines which would help the victims fight the virus loads. No targeted medicines were in place to treat the patients. Yet some drugs were reassigned to manage the disease as a loosely constructed remedy, which, however, became popular. Some businesses flourished on this arrangement.

Rumours and propaganda jammed social media, terrifying people, and benefiting the jacks. A free society became a controlled society. People were unable to move out of their homes. Neighbours were at an unseen distance. In historic times, that is how people lived under tyrants and thugs. The situation also resembled the heavy bombing during wartime where people had to stay indoors in fear and without food. Covid-19 contributed to economic devastations faced by laymen and had inexplicable and ongoing social damage on children.

According to India's most recent census conducted in 2011, there are 456 million migrants in India, representing 38% of the total population. The pandemic has had a severe impact on these individuals, many of whom rely on daily wages to support themselves and their families. The shutdown of various industries due to the lockdown has left these workers without any income, making it difficult to pay for basic necessities like food and shelter. The Government of India has not issued any guidelines mandating these industries to provide labourers with accommodation or food.

Migrants have been greatly affected by this crisis and often work in jobs where they are not paid well and have no benefits or security.

Some sections like sex workers had no source of income and were treated as an outcaste. No one showed sympathy, and life became bizarrely miserable for them.

According to the National AIDS Control Organisation, a division of the Ministry of Health and Family Welfare, there are approximately 9 lakh female sex workers in India. Additionally, data gathered from 17 states shows that 62% of the 62,137 transgender persons engage in sex work as well. However, sex work has come to almost a complete halt since March 2020 because the pandemic has hit this community hard in a variety of ways. Sex workers in India are facing everything from debt and depression to the risk of contracting COVID-19.

Many rural and tribal people were receiving kits and basic assistance from the government in many ways. But this section of people, especially women, were deprived of care and respect from society. They were not enrolled for any privileges from the government.

The lack of relief made it especially difficult for sex workers, who were already in a precarious situation with no state-sanctioned safety net or family support. Their families often depended on their daily earnings just to get by, and they didn't have any savings or access to loans and other financial institutions. Public sector banks would routinely refuse loans to sex workers since they had no one to stand surety for them.

Private money lenders often take advantage of sex workers by lending them money at high-interest rates. This can quickly lead to a debt burden, as sex workers often don't have a regular income. This can then have a domino effect, making it difficult for sex workers to access other necessities like housing. Most sex workers who run single-headed households live in rented accommodation, and during the lockdown period, many have been asked to pay rent or vacate their homes.

The most visible and severe impact of the pandemic has been on necessities like food security and good nutrition.

The pandemic has hit necessities like food security and good nutrition the hardest. Sex workers were largely excluded from government-provided food relief packages, so they had to depend on food relief provided by non-governmental organisations (NGOs) and individual philanthropists. This didn't provide them with enough of the right kind of food to meet their needs, especially for HIV-positive sex workers, older sex workers living with comorbidities and pregnant women in sex work.

This is because the government didn't consider them as a part of society ever. Post-pandemic too earning has been a difficult task for them. Sex workers provide crucial but unexplained service in society, although no one accepts their work as a recognised service. They meet the physical needs of humans and indirectly keep a lot of undue crime under control.

Some states in India accepted such groups or their dwellings officially to run and render services, allocating them a specific location like the Kamathipura or in their identity of Red Street. But Kerala and many other states seem to have not bothered about the activities of such groups. Many governments have not recognised them for any privilege. So, they were not eligible for any government grants which were given to helpless or needy groups in society.

The pandemic left behind many lessons and underlined human failures in every sphere where scientists made claims of breakthroughs and achievements.

Nature didn't create anything uniformly for easy understanding by the human senses. Person-to-person difference has proven to be unbridgeable. When vaccines come, drug makers feel threatened and when people find their natural way to build immunity, the vaccine businesses feel threatened. When diseases spread like wildfire, drug makers are happy. When people are healthy, drug makers are unhappy. The vicious circle never stops. It has been proven that the nature of viruses and their pathogenic character is not perfectly determinable. As the nature of Covid-19 virus kept camouflaging, scientists fell into a deep delusion. Nevertheless, every challenge has a common remedy - that emerges from wisdom, that human sense is seemingly yet to attain. When the virus camouflaged, we chased it blindfolded wearing a mask and leaving space for incomprehensible devastations. The chasm between Before Corona (BC) and After Disease (AD) is too big to bridge, throwing a generation into doom.

Chapter 30

Bringing Ayurveda into the Picture

The stream of traditional medicines is catching up after finding their effectiveness. Since Covid-19 remained largely in cities and among those who follow the modern lifestyle, it is time to think about how the rural population was largely safe from the infection. It is their lifestyle! India's rural lifestyle still has a touch of traditional medicines, thanks to the influence of herbs in daily life through food and personal care.

But over a period, because of the gradual decline in doctors' expertise, knowledge of traditional medicines, and our option to reduce dependence on traditional medicines, we opened the way for modern medicines. As a result, modern medicines could rapidly invade the space of traditional medicines.

Now there are more medicines, more diseases, and more drug-related deaths. Here Ayurveda is the last hope.

Covid-19 has boosted acceptance of Ayurveda among people. Although, it happened after reluctance. Thanks to the government's initiatives in bringing Ayurveda into the limelight. Nevertheless, it seemed, the

Government of India was over-cautious of giving open support to Ayurveda, because of its fear of the antagonists' misinterpretation of its blind support to some giant Ayurveda-cum-OTC-cum FMCG companies.

Modern medicine practitioners were furious about the government's support for Ayurveda, as their medical association responded unpleasantly to the government's decision on declaring a protocol for Ayurveda in managing Covid-19.

The advocates of the first-line treatment, modern medicine, did not want to accept the rear-line. Practitioners of modern medicine have always been vociferously against traditional medicine. Modern medicine liked to call India's traditional medicine a sample, or fake medicine. At the same time, they used to prescribe many medicines prepared on Ayurvedic bases, packed as modern medicines, and sold by pharmaceutical companies. In many cases, the so-called sample delivers better and lasting results, which are naturally desirable for human beings.

Under classical Ayurveda, there were powerful medicines, which are rarely available for people's benefit, because of their hyper-commercialisation. Most people have been found to take resort to Ayurvedic preventive medicines and other home care remedies in line with traditional medicines.

Indian life is deeply and irreversibly connected with traditional medicines. Most people in India consume turmeric, pepper, ginger, jeera and many herbs and spices with medicinal values almost daily. Most Indians in their vicinity have tulsi and other herbs, which are good for one or the other disorders. They are familiar with numerous Ayurvedic immunity boosters, which are commonly available in medical and provision stores. People are aware of the advantages of Ayurveda in daily life. These practices build their immunity and save them from normal cough and cold syndrome.

Many people understood the strengths of Ayurveda for the first time in the days of Covid-19. Even those who are practicing modern medicines advised their patients to follow traditional home remedies. Although they were shy of openly accepting the truth about Ayurveda's healing potential.

Death by virus happened not because of the lethality of the virus alone. Many of the deaths happened because of co-morbid issues and contradictions of the non-targeted medicine used for the treatment. The fraternity of modern medicine may not accept the mistake, even though they may not be able to say how safe the medicine they used for the treatment of severe cases was. Many shreds of evidence suggested that the deaths and consequent panic have been the result of the wrong treatment protocol suggested by WHO, and the adoption of the same blindly by the infected countries. Most Covid-19 deaths were because of trials carried out on patients by doctors with medicines, launched by pharmaceutical companies claiming the same as remedies. Shockingly, these medicine manufacturers could successfully procure a licence to sell these medicines in various countries at various times. The sellers of these medicines could influence the change in treatment protocol according to their business interests. More than 90 per cent of the infections were treatable at home, as we see these days, given the rate of recovery reported daily. More than three-fourths of the cases did not need any medicine, but traditional home remedies.

Covid-19 deaths were not just deaths by illness, but a genocide on patients by pharmaceutical companies under the blessing of modern healthcare systems, WHO showed lopsided approaches towards the regulatory authorities of infected countries. Many allopathic practitioners, who did not wish to be quoted, confirm that the concerns were escalated by many missteps. A viral infection is just a common disease. For some patients, it becomes critical when pneumonia sets in with the viral infection leading to inflammation of the airspaces in the lungs. Pneumonia is usually more dangerous for people over 65 years.

Allopathic treatments completely transformed from a symptoms-based approach to a test-based approach, even if the illness was rightly presumable. This added to the burden on patients. Indeed, a capitalist-driven modern healthcare system cannot be different in its approach.

Chapter 31

Loka Samastha Sukhino Bhavantu

India needed an integrated healthcare approach for tackling the pandemic that would surely be an endemic health crisis. There was a big challenge in managing drug-induced healthcare complications, ensuring affordable treatment, and better health of citizens with the support of indigenous medicine. Post-pandemic, people lost their trust in modern medicines and modern medicine practitioners because of business motives. People are looking at traditional medicines for immunity boosting to resist infections. Things have begun to change. We can only hope that the spirit of the government in taking indigenous medicine to a desirable level remains intact, without giving in to the pressure of lobbies of modern medicine.

We are all bound to live by the order of nature, as other beings live in nature. For curing ailments too, we need to look at nature's resources. We were unable to take home the benefits of traditional medicines, even in the days of the pandemic. We have left the great legacy of life science behind the bunged history and chosen to crosscut our way to acquire the knowledge that has incidentally been succinct. Other streams of medicine like Homeopathy also had solutions.

The preventive medicine also reportedly worked well. Even though the advocates of modern medicine used to call traditional medicines placebo, Ayurveda and Homeopathy rendered admirable results.

There were instances of Ayurvedic doctors successfully treating Covid-19 cases with multiple complications. The medical fraternity, dominated by modern medicine practitioners, rarely acknowledged such successful instances. At the official level also, the strength of Ayurveda was not recognised. Ayurveda, with all its sense of responsibility and social commitment, had contributed modestly, but greatly, to our country's fight against the pandemic.

The first Indian case of SARS-CoV-2 infection was reported from Kerala, and since then, the state government has been on high alert to handle any potential crisis. With a considerable inflow of COVID-19-positive persons from other states and countries during the early phases of the pandemic, Kerala implemented an active COVID-19 containment strategy.

In response to the outbreak, the state increased its contact tracing, testing, and tracking efforts to flatten the curve and relieve pressure on hospitals. The state health department stressed the importance of following Covid-appropriate behaviour, such as social distancing, wearing masks, and proper hand sanitising. The protocol followed in Kerala is done under guidelines issued by the Federal Government and WHO protocols.

These guidelines are systematically updated based on new research and findings. In addition to accepted pharmacological and non-pharmacological interventions, traditional medicines (Ayurvedic medicines) were also used to boost the innate immunity of individuals and to manage early uncomplicated cases of COVID-19 infection, as an adjunct to conventional management protocols.

The therapeutic benefits of using Ayurvedic management for infectious diseases in Kerala were not fully documented, though the treatment is generally well-accepted and provided through public and private Ayurvedic dispensaries and hospitals.

Although there are 947 public Ayurvedic healthcare facilities in Kerala, they are only managed by 1,500 Ayurvedic doctors with a bed strength of 3,154. This lack of resources resulted in an inferior service delivery system when compared to the general health system.

In the early phase of the pandemic, the Government of Kerala (GOK) constituted a seven-member Task Force to prepare the blueprint of an Ayurvedic strategy for the prevention and mitigation of COVID-19. GOK thereafter approved a comprehensive organisational algorithm and an action plan for implementing the strategy.

In the early phase of the pandemic, the Government of Kerala (GOK) constituted a seven-member Task Force to prepare the blueprint of an Ayurvedic strategy for the prevention and mitigation of COVID-19. GOK thereafter approved a comprehensive organisational algorithm and an action plan for implementing the strategy. This action plan included having designated hospitals for COVID-19 patients, setting up a 100-bed facility at an Ayurvedic hospital in Kochi, and starting an intensive training programme for doctors and health workers on the use of Ayurvedic medicines for COVID-19.

The Ayush Department created a structured participatory model before implementation, with the active involvement of various Ayurvedic professional organisations and local self-governments (LSG's). An essential drug list was also approved for the prevention and mitigation of COVID-19. This was done by collating the opinions of over 300 Ayurvedic experts and taking inputs from the guidelines of the Health Department, GOK and Ayush Ministry, Government of India.

Various Ayurvedic Programmes for the COVID-19 Pandemic

From the onset, the GOK implemented various Ayurvedic Preventive Strategies (APS) to strengthen the innate immunity of the public against COVID-19. The strategy covered different categories of the population based on age and risk of exposure. These were Swasthyam (which means good health) for the general population below 60 years, Sukhayushyam (which means healthy old age) for the general population above 60 years, and Amritham (which means nectar) for the Covid-quarantined population.

The strategy of Punarjani (which means rejuvenation) is intended to ensure a speedy return to normal health in individuals in the post-Covid phase without any lingering Covid sequel. Further, the government implemented the Bheshajam (which means free from disease fear) programme, providing Ayurvedic treatments to asymptomatic or mildly symptomatic COVID-19 patients who had given consent for the same.

On the other hand, modern medicine manufacturers made a fortune on the supply of exorbitantly high-cost medicines that killed many and left many with complications due to exposure to drug toxicity. Modern drugs have made our country the world's biggest market for lifestyle diseases. Every day thousands die of drug-induced organ failures and drug resistance. Indigenous medicine has a long history of effectively rescuing our country from the disreputation of being the biggest lifestyle disease market and saving humanity. Traditional Indian medicine is catching up now, and there is still some hope.

For a densely populated country like ours, if indigenous medicine is given due recognition and support, people will have easy access to affordable, more effective, and holistic health solutions. Covid-19 wouldn't have been so distressing had indigenous medicine too been brought to the limelight in the same manner allopathic drugs were given importance. We need an integrated approach tapping the strength of modern medicine and the full strength of indigenous medicine. Ayurvedic doctors believe that with the support of cutting-edge allopathic solutions also, people can be served with sustainable medical solutions.

Unfortunately, now indigenous medicine is not shaped into an organised stream as the systematic modern world requires. The improper education system and lack of good practitioners have further reduced the ingenious of nature's valuable healthcare system.

Indigenous medicine can contribute greatly to India's healthcare system. I hope our Indian government would integrate indigenous medicine with modern medicine without being inclined to the latter's market share and dominance. Indigenous medicine could undoubtedly be a natural, most reliable, and safe remedy for everyone against the pandemic.

Loka samastha sukhino bhavantu (May All Beings Everywhere Be Happy and Free) is India's prayer. To achieve it, we need a healthcare system keeping Ayurveda at the forefront and in line with modern medicines. It's high time we understand not to do blind following of only modern medicine but accept Ayurveda too as a way of life.

Chapter 32

WHO Defines

Complementary Medicine

The terms 'complementary medicine' and 'alternative medicine' refer to a broad set of healthcare practices that are not part of that country's own traditional medicine and are not fully integrated into the dominant healthcare system. They are used interchangeably with traditional medicine in some countries.

Conventional Pharmaceuticals

Conventional pharmaceuticals are defined as medicinal drugs used in conventional systems of medicine to treat or prevent disease or to restore, correct, or modify physiological function.

Herbal Medicines

Herbal medicines include herbs, herbal materials, herbal preparations and finished herbal products that contain active ingredients, parts of plants, other plant materials or combinations thereof. In some countries, herbal medicines may contain, by tradition, natural organic or inorganic active ingredients that are not of plant origin (e.g., animal, and mineral materials).

Indigenous Traditional Medicine

Indigenous traditional medicine is defined as the total of knowledge and practices, whether explicable or not, used in diagnosing, preventing, or eliminating physical, mental, and social diseases. This knowledge or practice may rely exclusively on experience and observation handed down orally or in writing from generation to generation. These practices are native to the country in which they are used. The majority of indigenous traditional medicine has been practiced at the primary healthcare level.

Chapter 33

Many Answerless Questions

The questions about the origin of the virus would never be answered because it was first reported in a city in China, at its famous virology lab. The world would only keep guessing until the memory of the pandemic flees the public someday. The WHO team would continue to grope in the dark, as China is unlikely to give the necessary details. Nonetheless, neglect of these questions would pose a serious challenge to human life on the planet.

In the beginning, everyone thought it might take some time for the world to adjust to the post-pandemic change. But changes have been rapid as people began to return to their normal life under compulsion, braving many months of fear. At the same time, we must remember, a generation's habits hardly change. If people felt fear at one time, they would return to their old habits once the fear subsides. No fear is permanent. No habit is changeable unless one decides to consciously change. During the pandemic days, people rapidly changed their mindset and lifestyle for some time and learned to live within tight corners.

At least some might have thought of living sustainably with the circumstantially forced changes. Most people started washing their hands once they returned home, and before touching anything. People started taking baths using more soap, which might have pushed India's otherwise lower per capita consumption of toilet soap. But there is a concern about the change in the habits of jobless youngsters and students. The most fearful thing might be the loss of discipline in their routine life. That is no less than a social disaster.

On the other hand, the steep rise in sales of sanitisers and its subsequent fall reflects the change in human habits.

If people could learn anything for a desirable change, that would be a good sign. Nevertheless, we need to be cautious about many things that could destroy the new world order. The forces that exploited the masses at the time of the pandemic would continue to wield their influence and become richer at the cost of people's misfortune. The opportunities to exploit will only keep the habit more active. That means further exploitation.

Then there is a genuine question. Will this be the 21st century's last pandemic or will it lead to a more frequent outbreak of epidemic?

The pandemic makes some business sharks richer at the cost of the laymen's trouble. Research and Development (R&D) activities are undoubtedly admirable. Biotechnology will continue to play a major role in the days ahead as a big contributor to business growth. And when these research findings contribute to building a business and creating a new market to thrive on sickness, a frequent outbreak of pandemic might be a regular event. Let us not forget, almost every century saw a pandemic. Some of them are endemic. We are only 2 decades into the 21st century and have already been hit by one pandemic. The pandemic was active for more than a year until people and the government began to consider the situation as normal, even without stopping the count of infections.

People may now remember, for the first 15 months, the entire human world stood on its toe as a viral particle tested all human achievements – social, economic and scientific. Covid-19 exposed modern medicines' dark side and questioned all treatment protocols. Astonishingly, the world continued to tighten the calibration of the medical approach. The quality of medical care deteriorated steadily. Simultaneously, modern medicine has been unable to justify its conclusion about the nature of viruses.

When the infection broke out, it was said to have originated from bats. Later, it seemed the bat origin theory seemed to have been abandoned by scientists. Many theories emerged subsequently. The entire world suspected where the infection originated, Wuhan has a virology institute named, Wuhan Institute of Virology (WIV). After the pandemic broke out, the virology institute became a centre of controversy. As the world was about to settle on the fear of the pandemic, WHO sent a team of investigators to visit the heavily guarded Wuhan Virology laboratory, apparently the assumed place of origin. The team visited the premises to ascertain some clues about the origin of the virus. Here they spent less than 4 hours and discussed with the well-known virus hunter 'Bat Woman' named Dr Shi Zhengli of WIV. And this is what the media news report quotes of the WHO team's visit to WIV.

"Most scientists, including Shi, rejected the hypotheses of a lab leak. However, some experts speculate that a virus captured from the wild could have been figured out in a lab experiment to test the risks of a human spillover and then escaped via an infected staff member. She had initially expressed fear that the virus could have leaked from the lab, according to an interview with Scientific American. Later, checks showed that none of the gene sequences had matched the viruses that staff members were studying. Some scientists have called for China to release details of all virus samples studied at the lab, to see which most closely resembles SARS-CoV-2."

The outside world had all the reasons to suspect that the virus was leaked from the lab, though China repeatedly silenced all allegations. Interestingly, one of the team members, Dominic Dwyer, an Australian expert in infectious diseases said, China refused to give raw data on early Covid-19 cases to the WHO team probing the origin of the virus. Circumstantially also, there were enough reasons to suspect China. With good expertise in manoeuvring and taking the world for a ride, China always tries to succeed in its game. Given the history of China's penchant for keeping secrecy, it is not very easy for anyone to gatecrash into the secrecy of their lab. Like the world, powers could not do anything in the arms-making case of Iraq under Saddam Hussein when there was suspicion of its work on biological weapons.

A strenuous search for the virus' origin may not take the world a long way. China has enough with it to drive WHO towards where it desires. The lab authority, before the WHO team visit, had offered various explanations and said it could isolate only 3 closely related live bat viruses which were related to SARS that broke out in 2003. The world has no option but to believe what China projected.

To one of the questions asked by the science magazine Shi Zhengli, a Chinese scientist who led a group that studies bat coronaviruses at the WIV answered: "According to the findings of our team and our international peers, SARS-CoV-2 is very likely to have originated from bats. It may have evolved one or more intermediate hosts, become adapted to humans, and eventually spread among humans."

"However, it remains unclear which animals were the intermediate hosts and how they spilt over to humans." Since then, various theories have emerged, besides too many contributions from professionals and amateur medical commentators through social media. Constantly changing medical arguments and many inconsistencies. In conclusion, healthcare regulators are puzzled by all this; ultimately, a huge cost was paid by human beings with their wealth and life. The embattled human beings finally gave in to their defeat and stood ready to settle with huge losses of wealth and time.

I am sure, the scientific world may not be interested in such an expedition since the pandemic has opened new opportunities for vaccine developers. Though vaccine developers' challenges are not going to be over so quickly. Anything that was done in a hurry, without allowing nature to process it, will collapse like a fort built with sand.

The Global Corruption

The novel coronavirus, while still wreaking havoc and causing death, has also brought to light different forms of corruption that have contributed to weakening healthcare systems. According to reports, in the first 10 months of the pandemic, more than 1800 people contacted Transparency International's Advocacy and Legal Advice Centres to report Covid-19-related corruption cases.

Nemexis, a Berlin-based anti-fraud consulting firm, found that corruption in healthcare services weakened healthcare delivery in 58 countries surveyed, contributing to Covid-19 deaths in every third country.

Since the start of the outbreak, governments loosened their regulatory environment to expedite their Covid-19 responses. Covid-19-related corruption in service delivery caused dire effects on groups who were most reliant on health and other public services, such as women, poor people, and people from migrant/ethnic backgrounds.

The pandemic has increased the pressure on healthcare procurement to be transparent. Transparency International found that, during the initial months of the pandemic, governments purchased some goods at 25 times the original price. A survey run by the International Federation of Accountants confirmed evidence of fraud, corruption, and mismanagement of public funds that created a sense of urgency among many people. The relaxation of checks and balances, increasing demand, and shortages of essential medicines, PPE, ventilators, and medicines caused a strain on global supply chains, making them more vulnerable to corruption.

Here are some corruption cases documented worldwide by CMI, an anti-corruption resource centre-

- Ministers and vice-ministers in Peru, Ecuador, Bolivia, and Panama were implicated in corruption cases and forced to resign.
- Somalia took 4 high-level health officials to court over allegations of misappropriating pandemic relief funds.
- High-level political leaders and wealthy individuals in Canada, Peru, Argentina, Spain, and Poland have jumped the queue to access Covid-19 vaccines.
- Zimbabwe's Minister of Health was arrested over alleged corruption related to the awarding of a USD 60 million contract for Covid-19 supplies.

These and many more corruption stories came to light when people were just about getting to know the virus and dealing with the unprecedented changes it brought to nationals worldwide.

Data manipulation is one of the key signs of corruption during the COVID-19 pandemic, according to Transparency International. This can lead to devastating consequences, including misallocation of resources, spikes in case rates as citizens unaware carry on as normal and increased mistrust in governments when reality does not match the official version of events.

Studies based on rates of the population with COVID-19 antibodies have suggested that SARS-CoV-2 is more prevalent in many countries than official statistics reveal. This data manipulation can have devastating consequences, such as the misallocation of resources and increased mistrust in government agencies.

According to a 2020 report by the World Bank review, several new threats will usher post-lockdown and impact by -

Rising Economic Downturn

The restrictions implemented to help manage the virus and its effects have had a profound impact on economic growth.

Impact on Businesses and Jobs

The pandemic has taken a toll on businesses and jobs around the world. Many companies, especially micro, small, and medium enterprises in developing countries, are struggling to stay afloat. More than half of them are already behind on their bills, and many more are likely to fall into arrears shortly.

The economic fallout from COVID-19 will continue to put human capital at risk as families experience reduced incomes from job loss, cuts in remittance payments, and other factors.

The High Cost of Health Care

The outbreak of COVID-19 has made it evident that there is a worldwide need for accessible and affordable healthcare. This pandemic has affected countries in many ways, but one of the most significant ways is through human capital.

Closing Classrooms

According to UNESCO, at the height of the COVID lockdown, more than 160 countries had mandated some form of school closures, impacting 1.5 billion children and youth worldwide. The long-term effects of COVID-19 on education could be felt for decades to come, causing not just a loss of learning in the short term but also diminishing economic opportunities for this generation of students.

Gender Distinctions

The novel coronavirus presents a real and serious threat to other development divides such as the gender gap. The pandemic was responsible for reversing the decades of progress for women and girls in terms of human capital, economic empowerment, and voice.

Millions More Without Meals

Children, both male and female, are especially vulnerable to the global rise of food insecurity, which affects people living in both rural and urban areas. Beyond access to education, this rise in food insecurity puts children at risk for several health complications.

Fragility, Conflict, Violence: Home to More and More Poor

The COVID pandemic has enhanced the effects of fragility, conflict, and violence in many areas, threatening to reverse years of development progress.

Where did we go wrong in our calculations and estimations?

Let us count the deaths by comorbidities among Covid-19. Can any country appoint a Commission of enquiry to ascertain the cause of

Covid-19 deaths, to fix responsibilities of these killings? The world was unprepared to face the virally infectious pneumonia called Covid-19 that created havoc. As mentioned in the earlier chapters, one does not need a super brain to tell the plain truth about China's penchant for keeping secrets and fabricating its history. WHO learned about the virus much later, perhaps after China's feared a backlash from the rest of the world, by that time, Europe and America had begun to show their vulnerabilities towards the virus. It spread like a wildfire in countries where China, directly and indirectly, had its footprints. As many as 213 nations were hit.

Chapter 34

What is the Solution?

It is time to prove that Covid is nothing but a fear that someone has created. The media and Covid experts have their stake in this. Now the media lens is shut on this once-hot scoop. The topic has expired after an overdose.

A pandemic that took the world by storm is not serious now, experts believe. Virology as a system works only on weaknesses and faint immune systems. It's like killing poison with poison. Our system is controlled by viruses and bacteria, and we are a living abode for them. In such a scenario, we cannot be devoid of bacteria and viruses, and being extra protective, in fact, would lower our immune system. We as humans don't feel hungry, but the chemicals in our body is giving a message to process food, which is a requirement of our body's microbes and bacteria.

Viruses are omnipresent, and they are there in our bodies. Our body fights all viruses, of which we are not aware.

A lab can culture viruses. There are reasons to believe that all are human-created changes. Powerful viruses thrive on the consequent changes in weather conditions. Our scientists are experts in wonderfully naming all the virus variants. Let them continue to do it. The new variant will create trouble for humans and other species. We, humans, believe that all other lives on earth are generated for the stability of our ecosystem. So, we shouldn't care about how these viruses affect other species. We think only about ourselves and take cruel decisions for other species. When there is a spread of such viruses, we take full right to eradicate them just for our safety. Who has given us the power to kill other living beings?

Humans forget the fact that all these virus systems started to damage our lives because we are responsible for this situation as we interfere in their lives. The story started from the time we shifted our lives from forests to leading a better life. But we still want to go back to the forest, and we believe deep down that it belongs to us. The concerns about viruses started after we lost touch with naturalism, as we embraced modern life. This shift increased our vulnerability to diseases. In a way, we created these diseases and laid blame on innocent animals for bringing the viruses. We never tried to find a solution to heal them but mercilessly killed them when they carry any disease or infection. Humans have no value for other lives on earth.

For example, recently, the government cleaned up many pig farms in Kerala by brutally killing them after paying compensation to the owners. We can fill every hole with money. Interestingly, the caretakers were feeling bad for killing them and were ready to take utmost care. However, the experts feared that wild pigs could easily infect the farm pigs. The virus is harmless to wild animals. We are overlooking the truth by reading between the lines with suspicion.

All these matters are crystal clear; it is our greed and messy lifestyle that is the real villain. But we have no heart to accept the fact. We are smart enough to pass the buck to someone else.

Virologists count more than 10,000 dangerous viruses. These viruses can give us sleepless nights. Let us say if there are so many dangerous viruses, we will be under their attack daily. Then what will we do? What does our future look like? Perhaps, there will be a time when WHO will be tired of declaring health emergencies after emergencies.

Vaccination Compulsions

The Supreme Court refused to intervene in the plea demanding compulsory vaccination for the entire public. If the government makes it mandatory, the Court finds no room for its interference. At the same time, the permission for vaccinated people to travel on local trains has made 25,000 people living in Navi Mumbai ineligible for a ticket or season ticket. It seems the person sitting at the counter dictates rules. There is no standard regulation. The counter officials often deny tickets for essential travelling without an identity card of a government employee.

The decision of making 2 doses of vaccination compulsory could land many people in trouble. It is impossible to get it overnight. The decision should have a reasonably relaxing time. Covid shield requires an 85-day gap between the 2 doses. Even if a person wants to follow the government's decision, he has to wait for 86 days. A hasty worker with no capacity to have a paid jab has to suffer the tightrope for 3 more months. Free vaccines are not available easily without a godfather at the inoculation centres. Until the 2 doses are complete, the law forbids their presence in public places and the right to travel by train, as if they are criminals. But the jam-packed transport continues to throng the roads.

By the middle of August, the fully vaccinated people in Mumbai constituted only 20%. Out of this, only a few of them must be regular travellers for a livelihood. Initially, the government vaccinated only senior citizens. They do not travel for jobs. The active working-age population got it late. Even after the coverage of the lower-age category, many people were unable to take it due to the infection in the second wave that hit the younger population. An infected person cannot take the jab within 3 months. The infection rate among people who took the first jab was substantial. They could not take the second dose even 5 months after the first dose. Our health experts and policymakers did not assess the reality before embarking on an ambivalent policy.

- Doesn't the government want the vulnerable and unfortunate segment to work and earn their livelihood?
- What about unexpected deaths and negligence in the name of medicines and vaccines?
- How about the deaths because of the fear of the pandemic and living secluded?
- What about the health problems caused by masks?
- What about the wasted 2 years of children's academics?
- What about the trailing effect of exposure to electronic devices on the younger generation?
- What about the financial deficit people have encountered due to the loss of jobs, shutting down of businesses, and pay cuts due to Covid?
- What about losing a loved one because of the negligence and unpreparedness of the authorities?
- What about 2 years of progress stalled in the name of lockdown?

Contradictions never end. The 2 strict lockdowns hadn't rendered any result. Neither did the lockdown stop migrant workers from moving to their native place nor did the so-called farmers stop sittings in the streets. Elections came and went like carnivals. The crowd size was never thin.

A whole house has been burned to kill the lizard on the girder. The purpose wasn't achieved. The burned house bears the face of a ghost. Yet we laugh it off. That is how we can summarise the terrific mismanagement of the Covid-19 pandemic.

Chapter 35

How the World Leaders Responded to Covid-19

Covid-19 was notoriously hard to control, and political leaders were only part of the calculus when it came to pandemic management. But some current and former world leaders have made little effort to combat outbreaks in their country, whether by downplaying the pandemics' severity, disregarding science, or ignoring critical health interventions.

This lack of effort has been costly in terms of lives lost and economic damage done. Inaction in the face of a global pandemic is like negligence for the choices the leaders made.

Narendra Modi of India

India was the new epicentre of the global pandemic, recording some 400,000 new cases per day by May 2021. The country's health minister proclaimed in March that the pandemic was reaching an 'endgame.' However, Covid-19 was gaining strength in India and worldwide—

but his government made no preparations for possible contingencies, such as the possibility of a deadlier and more contagious Covid-19 variant.

Although some areas of the country were still struggling to get the virus under control, Modi and others in his party held large outdoor campaign rallies before the April elections without taking precautions like wearing masks or social distancing. Additionally, he allowed a religious festival that attracts millions of people to go on from January to March without cancellation or postponement. Public health officials now believe this festival may have been a super spreader event and resulted in many new cases of the virus.

Carlo Borghetti, Italy, The vice-premier of Lombardy

"For the past 20 years, the region invested heavily in hospitals, which are now among the best in Europe. Unfortunately, they did not make the same investment in local health services: health clinics, rehab facilities, community nursing and family doctors. And as a result, they drowned much more than other countries in the pandemic."

Caro said, "We made a mistake by admitting patients infected with COVID-19 into hospitals throughout the region."

"We should have set up separate structures immediately for people sick with coronavirus, to not send COVID patients into healthcare facilities that were still uninfected. The biggest mistake we made was admitting patients infected with COVID-19 into hospitals throughout the region."

Jair Bolsonaro of Brazil

Bolsonaro's shoddy management of the pandemic has led to infighting within his government. Brazil has had 4 health ministers in less than a year. The country's uncontrolled outbreak of the virus has given rise to new variants, including the P.1, which appears more contagious.

Alexander Lukashenko, Belarus

Alexander Lukashenko has been the long time authoritarian leader of Belarus. He has never openly acknowledged the threat of Covid-19. At the beginning of the pandemic, as other countries were imposing lockdowns, Lukashenko chose not to implement any restrictive measures that would help prevent the spread of Covid-19. Ironically, he claimed that drinking vodka, visiting the sauna, and working in the fields would be enough to keep the virus at bay. His denial left the preventive measures and pandemic aid totally up to individuals and crowdfunding campaigns.

Donald Trump of the United States

Although Trump is no longer in office, the devastating long-term consequences of his mishandling of the pandemic continue to plague the United States - especially when it comes to the health and welfare of communities of colour.

From the beginning, Trump's denial of the pandemic, active misinformation about treatments and mask-wearing, and incoherent leadership damaged the country as a whole—but some groups were hit much harder than others. These big differences amplified existing problems such as poverty, housing instability, and the quality of schooling—and will likely continue to do so for a long time.

Trump's rhetoric surrounding Covid-19, which included racist terms such as 'Kung flu,' preceded a nearly two-fold increase in attacks against Asian Americans and Pacific Islanders in the past year.

Andrés Manuel López Obrador of Mexico

Mexico has the world's highest case fatality rate for Covid-19, with 9.2% of patients dying from the disease. It has suffered 617,000 deaths—on par with the U.S. and India, both countries with much larger populations.

A combination of factors has resulted in Mexico's prolonged, extreme Covid-19 outbreaks. One of these factors is inadequate national leadership.

Throughout the pandemic, Mexican President Andrés Manuel López Obrador has sought to downplay the severity of the situation in Mexico.

Epilogue

The corona pandemic was like a well-scripted and sponsored programme that was artfully and tactfully deployed. The execution of the plot has proven that human beings can be taken for a ride easily by clever and ruthless minds. Even animals, whom we consider inferior to us in terms of intelligence, try to resist when other animals or humans keep them under shackles for a long time. They also break the shackles when they are kept chained for so long a time.

A close observation of what happens around us and how wisely we have approached many issues that challenged our peaceful existence has thrown up a question wherein the answer also lies. Have we lost our common sense and pledged freedom to someone forever? Human beings are treated as donkeys by this certain fraternity that wishes to dominate them. Still, we humans faced it all and have been unresponsive. Even after a year of the pandemic, we remained docile and in control.

Tomorrow, if the government and media stop giving attention to the spread of the pandemic, will it be there to dominate our minds or manipulate us? Certainly not!! No one knew where the foul came from and ended, and no one would be there to take any responsibility. Nothing can compensate for the loss of one's life. No great achievements in the future can compensate for the loss suffered by mankind during the pandemic. It is all etched in history now.

A couple of deaths were horrifically pictured and exaggerated as a piling up of carcasses, enough to amplify a disaster. The reported scenarios in New York in the U.S. and Bergamo in Italy in early 2020 shattered the world. The world remained shell-shocked at the sight, and that led to global panic. Out of fear, country after country began locking down ruthlessly, containing their people, shutting factories, stopping livelihood activities, closing schools, and blocking expensively built roads, rail lines, and airport runways. The news about the virus's spread created fear and anxiety. The government's call for a lockdown created more panic and fear. The government couldn't foresee the profound agony that people were put to suffer behind closed doors all over the country and the globe.

The second wave devastated India, especially the young population in cities and villages. Overburdened medical infrastructure crumbled miserably. The reason attributed to this was the unexpected emergence of the second wave. As the second wave came, the third wave was also predicted, though the possibilities were less. People paid a hefty price for their lives. Most of the deaths happened due to the timely unavailability of treatments and over-dosage of reckless drug combinations. The ruination by the second wave in India made too big a picture in the western media. That could be a celebration time for the drug multinationals, which tested their products on thousands of freely available people (the assumed guinea pigs).

Deaths happen during non-pandemic times also. But none used to count the numbers. When counting happened, the numbers began to terrify the world. Initially, when India reported a death toll of over 4000, the global media ran big news. Such news appeared only as a Covid-19 highlight to amuse some sections of business. It was after the second wave that drug companies' therapeutic ventures gained speed. These companies, which were engaged in vaccine development, suddenly saw an opportunity as the world's second-most populated country began to reel in infection. The media pictures spoke about opportunities available in India rather than calling for aid. Death, be it the death of an old or infant, is a tragedy. Every life is precious. Exaggerated news about these tragedies could only overcast doom in the minds of people.

If there was a business gained out of the doomed heart of people, such business is more tragic than the pandemic itself. In a country where more than a billion people are struggling to live upon their lost opportunities, a tragic portrayal is only a crime against humanity. Our doctors also recklessly prescribed medicines in the name of cutting viral loads. There were incidents of prescribing both anti-bacterial and anti-viral drugs along with a heavy dosage of steroids. Side effects were also equally devastating. Incidents of blood coagulation and mucormycosis (black fungus) were seen rampant. Those who recovered from viral infection after heavy doses of drugs, for a long time had several imbalances noted in their biomarkers.

While some experts used to say such imbalances were only the reflection of the infection the patients suffered and did not need further medication to correct them, doctors commonly prescribed further medicines, which the patient's body couldn't sustain. These pointed out reasons for a probable relapse or side effects in the future.

They brought down the mortality rate, but most of the recovered covid-19 patients are yet sitting on a time bomb assembled by doctors who mishandled their cases according to the direction of medical companies. Although the treatment protocol was set by regulatory authorities, the protocol was only a façade. Inside the hospital, what the doctors did was a mystery at the cost of patients. Enraged relatives of patients called it a looting spree. In some states, with judicial intervention, the cost was capped. In the third wave, some experts announced children too were infected. This fear made people rush for the vaccine, making a safe landing for the vaccine business, considering India's child population.

All these sounded ridiculous. Rich countries like the United States and Italy didn't have enough facilities to cremate the dead ones and offer honourable last rites to the departed souls. In India, with very nominal numbers, the impact was avoidably and unreasonably overwhelming and that rendered only lifelong torments to millions of people. I personally witnessed the pain and suffering of innumerable people, and this was another compelling reason for this book. I chose to express my thoughts through letters, as I want people to never forget the devastating results of foul and human carelessness. We were careless where we needed to be prudent.

In human history, many epidemics devastated the world and redrew the borders of empires, killing millions from emperors to urchins and warlords to merchants. What was common was the sufferings of human beings, which were maybe to a lesser extent than what human beings suffered in the 2020-21 pandemic.

The pandemics of the earlier centuries were largely colonised and contained mainly in urban centres. Pandemic hardly crossed the boundaries. In the 21st century pandemic, the outspread of human suffering was beyond comprehending because of aggressive media coverage that created baseless panic. Foul minds of lawmakers, the vested interest of drug makers and shrewd healthcare providers also contributed to the ordeal. In India, it was during the time of Holi, 3 months after WHO alerted the world, the alarm first rang. Even after 3 months China first reported the virus, Indian borders remained wide open, and there was no report of any case. In all these months, there was a free flow of foreign traffic including from the infected cities of the world. Considering the rapidity of the virulence, a three-month time is a long period for beginning and spreading the infection. Nonetheless, the fire was lit very late, and some things could not be reversed.

I never stopped travelling. As an author and blogger would naturally discover a subject in what he sees, a traveller could see people on the move with their bags to faraway destinations. Unimaginable until then, the rare scene was not immediately understandable. A city like Mumbai had seen many disasters, but not as devastating as the lockdown. Not even the actual corona terrified the hapless people so intensely. We did the foolishness of a countrywide lockdown by simply following small urban-oriented countries. Large countries like the U.S. and China did not even follow the nationwide lockdown that India followed.

The Prime Minister of India said the Kurukshetra war ended in 18 days. He wanted 21 days from the public to fight the pandemic. The count was lost eventually. The life of 1.3 billion people steered through rough weather finding no recluse or anchor.

The decision to the lockdown was criticised. Unprepared was the excuse. There wasn't enough time to contemplate on preparation. There couldn't be any strategic reason for the all-of-a-sudden complete lockdown. The loss and sufferings of people at the cost of this humungous decision were far more severe than the Covid-19 toll and the infection itself. There could be nothing more painful than the worst experience of losing a dear one, with no last glimpses or even a decent final departure.

The survivors suffered the worst and will endlessly. The pandemic turned into an endemic eventually. It was a critical turning point in the history of humans, permanently having inscribed a mark of lost wisdom.

> *And the people stayed home. And read books, and listened, and rested, and exercised, and made art, and played games, and learned new ways of being, and were still. And listened more deeply. Some meditated, some prayed, some danced. Some met their shadows. And the people began to think differently. And the people healed. And, in the absence of people living in ignorant, dangerous, mindless, and heartless ways, the earth began to heal. And when the danger passed, and the people joined together again, they grieved their losses, and made new choices, and dreamed new images, and created new ways to live and heal the earth fully, as they had been healed.* – Kitty O'Meara

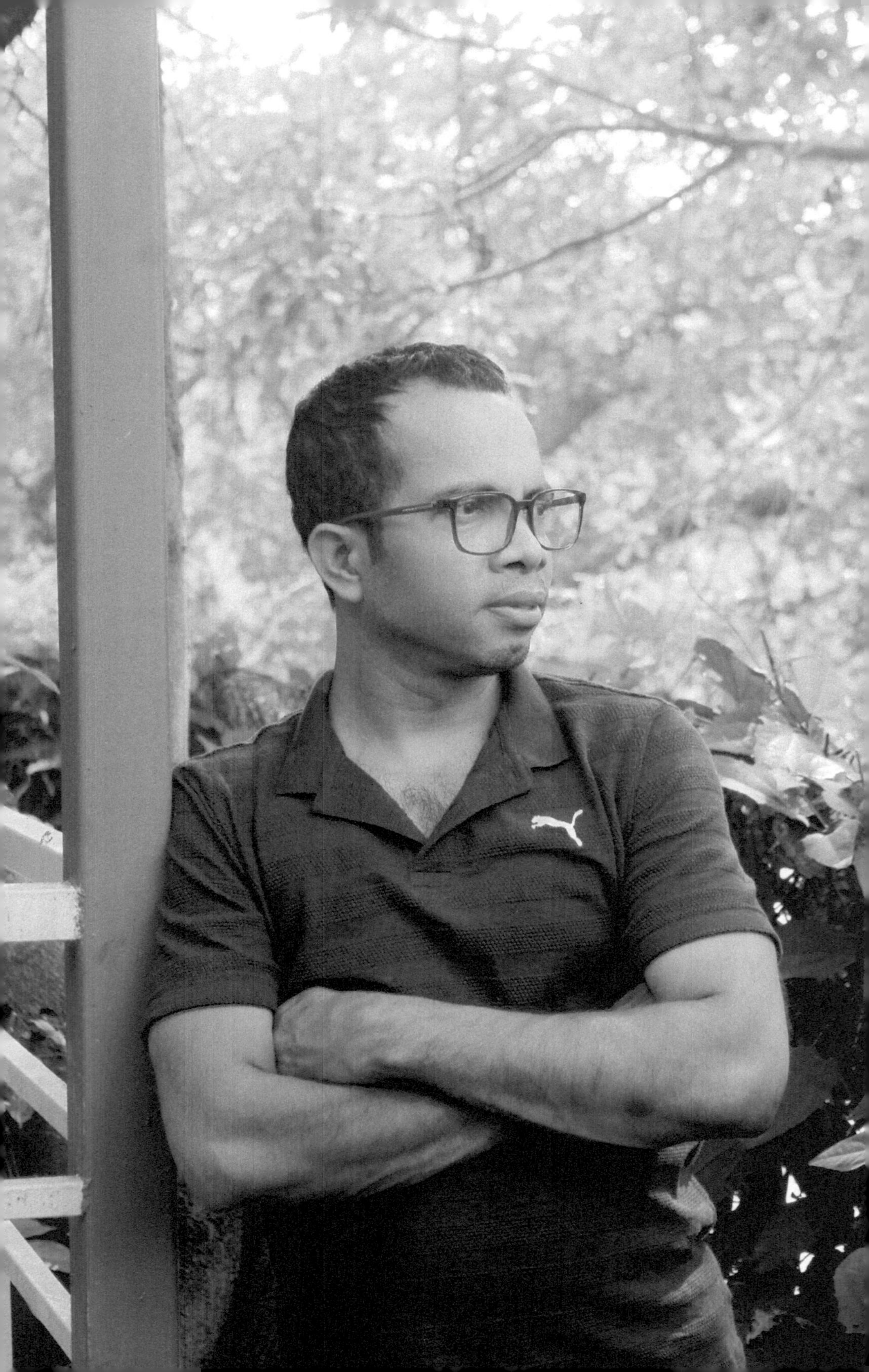

www.ingramcontent.com/pod-product-compliance
Lightning Source LLC
LaVergne TN
LVHW091310150826
845673LV00006B/1607

* 9 7 9 8 8 9 2 7 7 9 2 1 0 *